PENGUIN BOOKS

THE HOME STRETCH

Sanjay Dattatri is a software engineer. Over the last seven years, however, he has been working on various initiatives to make the lives of the elderly in India better. He was a full-time director of India's first store exclusively for senior citizens called the 'Old Is Gold Store', based in Chennai, for over five years.

He lives in Chennai with his wonderful and supportive wife, son and his mother-in-law. He can be reached at sanjay.dattatri@gmail.com.

T0158306

ADVANCE PRAISE FOR THE BOOK

'An invaluable guide for each one of us—at once educative and compassionate, born of the best of all teachers: serving those who cannot help themselves.'—Arun Shourie, Indian economist, journalist, author and politician

'*The Home Stretch*, a family caregiver's handbook written by Sanjay Dattatri, is a thoughtful and sensitive guide to caring for the sick and those with terminal health conditions. He delves into everyday issues of dealing with such an eventuality in your family and talks about its financial and emotional burden. Coming to terms with the fact that one needs to provide comfortable and clean care to a close relative while remaining sane and happy oneself calls for an organized approach that Sanjay so succinctly sums up. This is a guide that each of us could do with in our homes. A valuable insight into what to expect when a family member falls sick and how to deal with it on a daily basis.'—Leela Samson, dancer and choreographer

'Over the next few decades, we will see a robust growth in the population of senior citizens in this country. This book provides some valuable insights about caring for the elders in our families during their sunset years. Caring for elders needs to go hand in hand with compassion, such that they still feel they have a voice, and they have a role to play in their family and society. Sanjay has shared some very valuable insights based on his very personal journey.'—Meena Ganesh, CEO and MD, Portea Medical

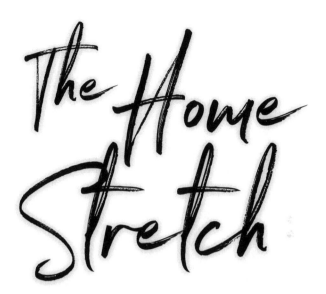

The Home Stretch

A Family Caregiver's Handbook

SANJAY DATTATRI

Foreword by Gopalkrishna Gandhi

PENGUIN BOOKS

An imprint of Penguin Random House

PENGUIN BOOKS

USA | Canada | UK | Ireland | Australia
New Zealand | India | South Africa | China

Penguin Books is part of the Penguin Random House group of companies
whose addresses can be found at global.penguinrandomhouse.com

Published by Penguin Random House India Pvt. Ltd
4th Floor, Capital Tower 1, MG Road,
Gurugram 122 002, Haryana, India

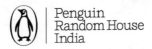

Penguin
Random House
India

First published in Penguin Books by Penguin Random House India 2021

Copyright © Sanjay Dattatri 2021

All rights reserved

10 9 8 7 6 5 4 3 2 1

The views and opinions expressed in this book are the author's own and the facts
are as reported by him which have been verified to the extent possible, and the
publishers are not in any way liable for the same.

ISBN 9780143452522

Typeset in Adobe Caslon Pro by Manipal Technologies Limited, Manipal

www.penguin.co.in

This book is dedicated to my mother, whose zest for life knew no bounds, and to my father, for having encouraged me to forge my own path.

Contents

Foreword   ix

Preface   xiii

Acknowledgements   xix

1. Fundamentals of Family Caregiving   1
2. Planning and Preparation   12
3. Bedridden Elder Care   25
4. Managing Hired Help   43
5. Managing Medication   55
6. Managing Hospitalization   64
7. Palliative Care and Beyond   78
8. Remote Caregiving   87
9. Managing Visitors   95
10. Taking Care of Yourself   106

11. Common Medical Equipment   117

12. Understanding Common Medical Procedures   135

13. Incontinence Management   146

14. A Safe and Secure Environment for Elders   162

15. Mobility and Accessibility   195

16. Retirement Communities   216

17. Importance of Sex and Companionship   235

18. Dementia Care   240

19. Activities for Seniors   253

Conclusion   259

Foreword

This book could be about you or me.

It is for you and me.

It is no easy read and yet, it has to be read.

It is about several truths, hard truths, written truthfully. I felt like skipping portions of the pre-publication draft while reading it because they were, for one at my stage of life, traumatizing. And—I must be truthful about a book that is so true—I did do exactly that. It was like averting one's eyes from a scene of pain. That exercise of skipping portions disentitled me from writing these words. But I felt Sanjay Dattatri will allow me the liberty when he reads the following sentence: I will read the book, if time and tide permit, from cover to cover, when it is published.

Time and tide.

This book is about something that is both unpredictable and utterly predictable. On the one hand, the medical conditions it describes with a clinical yet tender honesty are such that may never happen to one or to one's near and dear. *Touch wood!* On the other, they might have already started happening without our knowing it. Or they could happen at this very moment, even before I finish typing this line. *God forbid!* These two exclamations in italics are but human expressions. They may not be faulted by sober and mature minds. For who would want to be bedridden and immobile? And yet, that condition cannot always be wished away. It has to be faced and handled, should it arise. And faced and handled not just with love, but with competence.

The caregiver is not one at the beginning, but eventually has to become a professional. The hand that holds, cleans, grooms, feeds, clothes and administers medicine has to be strong, clean and adroit. And the mind that actuates that hand has to be Stoic. I use the word not just as a common adjective, but as a reminder of the Greek tradition of Stoicism in which the person following its tenets was able to face, with a cultivated indifference, pain and suffering (and equally, the opposites thereof). To be so deeply attached to the one being cared for and yet to steel oneself against the traumas involved is an almost superhuman requirement, and yet that is what is expected of the home caregiver. Nothing less can work.

A detached attachment is almost an oxymoron. And yet, that is precisely what this book tells us how to cultivate.

This book is a handbook, a guide and a manual, of course, but also so much more. It is sited on the margins of science and scripture. Does that sound 'too much'? Perhaps. But what, please tell me, can be more spiritual than 'help of the helpless'? That phrase is from the moving Christian hymn, 'Abide with Me'.

That is likely what the cared for is saying, wordlessly, or maybe even unawares, to the caregiver.

Gopalkrishna Gandhi
Bengaluru
13 July 2021

Preface

When my mother was seventy-seven years old, she was diagnosed with a rare neurological condition called Progressive Supranuclear Palsy—PSP for short. Not much is known about it, and there is no treatment available for it even today. It is a cruel disease, gradually robbing a person of all voluntary motor control while keeping the involuntary muscles, including the diaphragm, going strong, thereby keeping body and soul together interminably.

Over a period of two years, right in front of our eyes, she went from being an active, energetic woman to a completely bedridden patient, incapable of even moving her eyeballs. She remained that way for the next four years until she passed away at home early one morning.

As her condition was stable most of the time during this six-year period, barring a few hospitalization episodes, she remained at home under family care.

My brother was her primary caregiver. By virtue of being two streets away, I was one of the assistant caregivers on the weekdays and the primary caregiver during the weekends. A weekend warrior, if you will.

At that time, there was no single hospital with an appropriate multidisciplinary team that could help our mother's condition and so, for each specialization, we had to go to a different doctor in a different hospital. Doctors treated her as best as they could but didn't have the time or the patience to help us with caregiving at home.

Those were challenging times for all of us. As her disease progressed and her condition deteriorated, her faculties began to desert her one by one. First, she started losing her balance and her ability to walk independently. As a result, she fell down and broke her collarbone on one occasion. Then her speech problems started. It took her a lot of effort to put sentences together, and her words started slurring. Things escalated quickly after that and, two years in, she was unable to tell us if she was comfortable or in pain. In fact, from that time on, we were not even able to figure out whether she understood us but was unable to respond, or whether she could not understand us at all.

Needless to say, it was a traumatic experience for her and for us. We persevered gamely and over a period of time, we taught ourselves a lot about home healthcare. We scoured the surgical stores for products that could make her life better while also searching the Internet for information and guidance on caregiving. Gradually, through a process of trial and error, we learnt the art and science of family caregiving. For her part, during this entire period, our mother remained stoic and as accommodating and cooperative as she could be, given her condition.

Wanting to utilize this newfound knowledge for the greater good, a year or so after she was diagnosed, I quit my job as a software engineer and joined my friends to run India's first store exclusively for senior citizens, called 'Old and Gold Store'. The store sells over twenty-five different categories of products that can make life safe, secure and comfortable for active seniors as well as the bedridden. Equally usefully, the store provides guidance to new caregivers using our own hard-won experience.

While I provided advice and guidance to the customers, I also learned a lot from the unique experiences of the hundreds of people I met—doctors, physiotherapists, counsellors, nurses, administrators, senior citizens and, most importantly, other family caregivers.

This book is a humble attempt to collate all that knowledge into a lay person's guide to the challenging task of family caregiving.

For most of us, an unexpected event pushes us, with barely any notice, into the role of a primary caregiver. It is an experience that is akin to jumping into the deep end of a pool on the first day of our swimming lessons.

In recognition of that, I have structured the book to start at the deep end. The first chapter is an introduction. Once you have read through it, you will immediately find yourself in the thick of things. From Chapter 2 titled 'Planning and Preparation' to Chapter 11 titled 'Understanding Common Medical Procedures', I have written about how to take care of the bedridden elderly. Subsequent chapters deal with issues common to all elders, active as well as bedridden. The chapters towards the end are most relevant for caregivers and active elders.

The book can be read from beginning to end, if you so wish, but it can also be used as a reference book, as each chapter is independent of the others. In order to make the chapters standalone, I have written about some aspects of caregiving in more than one place. For example, you will find information (though not identical) on airbeds in three different chapters. This has been done expressly with the intent that the reader does not have to go back and forth in the book to gather all the details about the topic at hand. I hope this works as intended.

It is not a technical book and should not be mistaken for one written by a qualified medical professional, but it is the kind of book I wish I had had when we were looking after my mother.

I hope you find it useful. All the best to you and the loved ones you are looking after.

Acknowledgements

There are a lot of people who have been involved in the process of bringing this book out.

My mother was the inspiration for this book. It was her plight that first prompted me to look for such a book. Upon not finding one targeted at the Indian audience, I thought I might as well write one using the experience I had gained over a period of about seven years.

This book has been in the making for quite a while. Truth be told, it would not have seen the light of day if not for the constant goading and pushing by my wife, Gita S. Dattatri. In addition to this, she also read through all the drafts and made countless suggestions to improve the substance and structure of this book.

There were also many subject-matter experts who reviewed the various chapters of this book. I take this opportunity to thank Dr Kalaivani Ramalingam, Dr Ramesh Sadasivan, Dr Sridhar Vaitheswaran, Dr Chitrakala Rajkumar, Dr Anupama Rao and Manick Rajendran for their ready support and invaluable comments, corrections and suggestions.

My sincere thanks to my sister Aruna Kanchi and brother Shekar Dattatri for reviewing the book and helping me make it better.

The constant encouragement from my close friends, from the time I first voiced my idea for this book, has been a definite driving force. Without their regular enquiries, this book too would have ended up in my own special graveyard of unfinished projects.

Sincere thanks to my friend Sudha G. Tilak for her guidance and unstinting support. Special thanks to my dear friends, Prithvirajan and Jayashree, at the Old Is Gold Store. A shoutout to my wonderful gang in Udhavi.

A big thank you to the team at Penguin Random House India, including Manasi Subramaniam, Shiny Das, Shubhi Surana and Hina Khajuria for their support.

Finally, my thanks to the countless elders and caregivers I have had the privilege of meeting. This book would not have been possible if they had not shared their experiences with me so candidly.

Sanjay Dattatri
October 2021, Chennai

1

Fundamentals of
Family Caregiving

You are not alone

If you have recently started looking after an unwell loved one at home, then it is likely that you are beginning to believe that you are facing challenges that are uniquely your own and that you have been left all alone to tackle problems that you are ill-equipped to handle.

However, thankfully, that is far from the truth. Why thankfully, we will get to in a bit. The first thing to realize is that while you are in an extremely difficult situation, you are not alone in this predicament, given India's burgeoning senior citizen population. In all probability, there are literally hundreds of others around you, in your own town or city, who are going through much of what you are facing today.

Just to illustrate the diversity of problems faced by caregivers, here are a few examples. A seventy-year-old gentleman who, in an ideal world, should have someone looking after him, is taking care of his ninety-year-old mother all by himself. Another lady is looking after her husband, who is in his late seventies and suffering from late-stage Alzheimer's. In addition, she is also the primary caregiver for her mother-in-law who is close to a hundred, bedridden and, to top it all, refuses to eat. As a final example, there is a family of four octogenarians—a brother and three sisters—all unmarried and with no other close relatives, who live together and have to fend for themselves.

The number of examples of people having to face their own unique problems is endless. To paraphrase a well-known saying, 'each of the caregivers we meet has their own unique problems, just like every other caregiver'.

To look at it from a statistical standpoint, according to the UN Population Fund's India Ageing Report—2017, India is home to well over 10 crore senior citizens. Of these, an estimated 30 per cent suffer from some form of acute morbidity which prevents them from independently managing their own daily living activities. 8 per cent of the senior citizen population is living alone or with an equally old spouse. Finally, over 1 per cent, that is over 10 lakh elders, are bedridden or terminally ill, requiring round-the-clock care. In most of these cases, the primary caregiver for these people is a member of the immediate family, either the spouse or a child or, in some rare cases, a grandchild.

The fact that there are so many people who are going through or have gone through experiences similar to yours is a good thing (and hence the use of the word 'thankfully' before), because a great body of knowledge has been built up which can be of immense use to you. From tackling the common problems faced while looking after elders to ways of keeping your own identity and ensuring you get 'me' time without guilt, the collective wisdom of the millions before you can help and guide you through the days, months and possibly years of your caregiving life.

This book attempts to distil that knowledge into a few pages so that you have something to turn to every time you come across a new situation or issue.

What is caregiving?

Caregiving is the process in which one individual—the caregiver—looks after another individual—care recipient—who is in need of special support to get through their day. In the context of this book, the care recipient is an individual over sixty years of age with some form of disability.

Caregivers may be professional—nurses and nursing assistants—or family caregivers, meaning a member of one's immediate family, such as a spouse, child, son- or daughter-in-law, a grandchild or a close friend of the elder individual who needs the support.

In earlier times in India, professional caregiving was restricted to hospital stays only. All other caregiving was done at home by members of the extended family, all living together in a joint family system. In such large families, people of all age groups lived together and, between them, they managed to look after each other without too much stress accumulating on any one individual. Additionally, the fact that very few people lingered on for very long after any significant affliction meant that there were not that many long-term bedridden people around.

However, things have changed quite dramatically over the last couple of decades. On the one hand, the joint family system has all but disintegrated, especially in the urban areas, and on the other, the improving healthcare facilities available to everyone has increased longevity. Together, these two changes have increased the number of elders requiring home healthcare while simultaneously making caregiving a more difficult activity for the one or two family members who are around.

State of affairs in developed countries

In most developed countries, nuclear families have been the norm for many years now. Children move out of their parents' homes fairly early and lead independent lives. Old people also prefer to live independently and so, though we can still find cases of people looking after their unwell elder loved ones at home, more often than not, that job is assigned to professional care organizations such as old age homes, continuing care homes and palliative care centres. These organizations are professionally run, are monitored by umbrella organizations, and overseen by government departments and appropriate legislation. The personnel are usually properly qualified and well-trained to handle elders with different kinds of disabilities and needs, be it physiological or psychological.

Affordability of such facilities is, of course, an issue even in developed countries, but a combination of insurance, pension schemes, personal savings and welfare ensures that such facilities are accessible to the majority of the population.

Many of these developed countries have various organizations, both non-governmental and for-profit, that work for the benefit of elders. In America, for example, there is an association simply known as AARP that works to provide a better life to elders. Founded in 1958 as the American Association of Retired Persons, it is a membership-based NGO that is now one of the most powerful lobbying groups in the US with over 3.7 crore members.

Despite having such non-governmental organizations in addition to the federally funded Medicare, the problems are far from solved, even in an advanced nation like the US. Trends suggest that more and more people are choosing to be single and by 2050, a majority of Americans will be single, which will mean that many elders in the future will not even have a spouse to help them through their difficult days.

In Denmark, a socialist country, the government is completely responsible for the welfare of the elders. In the UK, the National Health Service (NHS) plays a big role in the care of elders, especially in areas related to medicine, while Age UK, a charity, looks into the welfare of seniors in multiple other ways.

In Japan, which has had a sizeable elderly population (around 20 per cent of their total population) for a long time now, the society is well-adjusted and geared up to take care of the elderly, and the quality of service is at an altogether different level. The culture of revering elders has not diminished in importance, and many of the companies famous outside Japan for electronic products (such as televisions and music systems), provide advanced senior-care products and services as well, which help to make the lives of the elderly safe, secure and comfortable. We need to look no further than Japan as a benchmark for high-quality elder care services.

Key differences in India

While developed countries adapted to changing demographics and brought in organizations, both private and public, to meet the needs of various segments of population, we in India, unfortunately dropped the ball when it came to supporting the elderly.

As we watched the joint family structure disintegrate, we did nothing to replace it with some other system that would take care of the ageing family members. We looked on with pride at the IT boom and the consequent migration of an entire generation of youngsters to different parts of the world, without thinking about what that would mean for the futures of their parents, the very people who were pushing their children to go and settle abroad.

Even today, believing our own mantra of 'India is a young country', we remain blind to the ever-growing greying population that has crossed 10 crore in number. Consequently, we find many people in their seventies and eighties living alone or with an equally old spouse in large, cumbersome houses that need constant maintenance and upkeep. Their children, of course, live halfway across the world, unable to do much more than call once in a while or send money over. With neither support nor security from family, the private sector or the government, these elders are leading a tough life.

Convenient retirement communities with senior-friendly homes and associated services are coming up only now and it will take a while before they mature and become capable of providing good-quality service.

Well-organized and well-equipped assisted living senior care homes and palliative care centres are practically non-existent. For love or money, it is hard to find a place where seniors with health issues can safely lead the rest of their lives in comfort without having to depend on their children and other relatives. Which brings us back to elders having to depend on their family for survival and protection.

Given that a majority of the seniors in India live at home, under the care of their immediate family, one would expect that there would be a lot of professional home healthcare agencies catering to this segment of the population. Alas, even here, the private sector and hospitals have been slow to react. There are only a few well-organized home healthcare agencies operating in India, and even these have only recently started to provide services, that too only in major cities.

A large number of local agencies do exist, but they are mostly unorganized, their personnel not very well-trained and some of the horror stories from people's dealings with them have to be heard to be believed. The largest requirement is not for trained nurses or doctors but for nursing assistants, who are unskilled or semi-skilled people capable of tasks such as changing diapers and helping with some of the daily living activities of the elderly. Unfortunately, there are but a handful of organizations working on identifying people capable of being nursing assistants, and even fewer organizations having the capability and capacity to provide a well-rounded training programme necessary to churn out the large numbers needed to meet market demands.

Hospitals seem to have their hands full with the services they already provide and hence are not always keen on adding home healthcare services to their portfolio. The doctors are not very enthusiastic either about leaving the comfortable confines of their clinics to make house calls, even if people are willing to pay them a premium for such a service.

Finally, there are not many organizations working for the betterment of the Indian senior citizens at a higher level. India does have a very broad, high-level national level policy on ageing under the Ministry of Social Justice and Empowerment. However, its implementation has been left to the individual states, which leaves a lot to be desired. HelpAge India and Dignity Foundation are a couple of organizations that are working in this sector, but their reach is still limited. Despite a majority of the politicians in India being senior citizens, one very rarely comes across any substantial action or meaningful discussions on ways to make India a senior-friendly country.

Professional caregiving and family caregiving

The bottom line is, you are likely to be doing most of the caregiving yourself, with some support from professional healthcare companies. A word of caution: the word 'professional' is used here only to differentiate these caregivers from family caregivers and should not be construed to mean that the level of service provided by them is necessarily professional.

Professional caregiving is a very nascent industry in India. As mentioned, doctors don't always have the time to make house calls, qualified nurses don't see it as a viable career path (for valid reasons) and the term 'nursing assistant' is just a politically correct way of referring to untrained personnel who don't have any other alternative means of earning a living.

However, that is not to say that nursing assistants are useless. Most people are intrinsically good and, with a little bit of training and oversight, can prove to be of immense help.

Therefore, as a family caregiver, you will have to use all your wiles, influence and clout to rope in professional caregivers as and when necessary to help you in your efforts. Every little bit of help will be needed along the way, and unless you are a doctor yourself—and even if you are—you will not be able to truly take care of your loved one without the help of other reliable professionals, such as doctors and nurses. So, as a first step, start by building contacts in your area so that you can call on necessary resources in an emergency. More on this later.

Physical, psychological and time demands

Nobody can say that caregiving is easy. Caregiving is going to take a lot out of your life—physically, emotionally, psychologically and in many other ways. On most days, you are going to be sleep-deprived, tired and enervated. You are going to constantly wonder if your loved one is comfortable and whether you are doing enough to keep them so. You are going to be wracked with guilt for not having taken some of the right decisions at the right times, even though they became obvious only in retrospect. On top of it all, watching a loved one wither and suffer at such close quarters is not going to make life easier. The sooner you reconcile to the fact that you will always feel this way, the better it will be for you in the long run.

However, that does not mean this is the end of your life. By realistically evaluating the situation, by sharing the burden of your responsibility with others, by understanding that you are untrained to take on this role and you can only do your best, and by understanding that you have a duty to lead a happy life for yourself, it is possible to escape the suffering described in the earlier paragraph—not entirely, but sufficiently to keep going.

2

Planning and Preparation

Taking stock

The first few days after you find out that your loved one is going to need special care can be a period of great turmoil.

If your loved one has been diagnosed with a neurological, degenerative disease such as Parkinson's, Alzheimer's or Progressive Supranuclear Palsy (PSP), the progression will usually be gradual, and this will allow you to accept reality and progressively take on additional tasks and responsibilities as required.

In contrast, an accident or a stroke can take a fully active person—someone who, until that moment, had probably been a rock for you in your life—and suddenly turn them into a completely dependent patient in an instant, forcing you to jump headlong into caregiving without warning, guidance or support. This period—during and just after hospitalization—can be as physically taxing as it is emotionally. The interminable waits in hospitals and having to deal with busy and overburdened doctors and nurses who don't have the time to sit and explain much to you can be quite trying.

Neither of these scenarios is easy to handle, and careful planning and preparation is required to manage the situation. From shock and worry, you have to move towards acceptance. From feeling all alone, you have to open your eyes and assess the available options for support and make the effort to reach out to friends and family. You have to face the reality and find answers to questions you don't want to even ask. Important questions like: How much money is this going to cost? Where is that money going to come from? Who can you enlist to help you? How will you manage the estate? How will you balance your career, your family, your life *and* this?

Sounds daunting and in many ways, it is. But once you have decided to grab the bull by the horns, things will get better.

Definitely.

Believe.

Acceptance

One day, medical science may succeed in helping us remain fit and young our entire lives. However, until that time, we have to live with an evolving discipline that is able to extend life, though it might not guarantee better health. With increased longevity and, consequently, an increasing greying population, it is inevitable that a good proportion of the elderly will need some level of special care during their last years. About 30 per cent of elders above the age of sixty suffer from acute morbidities, according to the India Ageing Report—2017 released by the UN Population Fund (UNFPA). Though there are no definitive numbers available, it is likely that about a third of these elders may be bedridden, needing round-the-clock support.

Life comes full circle for this group of bedridden elders. They become babies again, needing to be fed, cleaned, mollycoddled and have their diapers changed. The only difference is, babies grow up and provide multiple joyous occasions along the way. With the elderly, joyous occasions are few and there is no happy ending. The happiest endings are ones in which they pass away in their sleep without suffering from a long and lingering existence at the mercy of others. However, that is neither in your hands nor theirs.

If the loved one that you are looking after is terminally ill, the first thing you have to do is to accept the fact that death is inevitable. Your job is not to help them live forever, nor even to extend their life as long as possible. Your job, simply put, is to endeavour to provide the best care that is within your control to give so that they are comfortable and feel loved for as long as they are alive. Accept that there is only so much you can do.

If the care recipient is a parent, the onus of caregiving will invariably fall on one of the children and that might be you. Most caregivers, at some point in time, ask the question, 'Why me?' There is nothing wrong in asking that question, nor is it a sign of lack of love for the parent, so don't beat yourself over it if it pops into your mind unbidden. If circumstances have chosen you among your siblings as the primary caregiver, accept it. You can find ways to rope in the others as required and as the days go by, but for now you must accept that you are the chosen one.

Accept that you are probably not fully qualified and will never be to handle all the challenges that come your way. Accept that in hindsight, at least some of the problems you faced along the way could have been handled better. Accept that others may also think so—thanks to hindsight, obviously—and even go so far as to uncharitably say that if they had been in your shoes . . . well, they were not, were they? Accept that sometimes their criticism may be valid. Accept that it does not help to obsess over what could have been.

Accept that the care recipient may sometimes not appear appreciative of your efforts. People with advanced-stage dementia may not know what they are doing or saying. Even people whose mental faculties are largely intact may be irritable and uncooperative, sometimes. In their defence, just imagine how it must feel to be independent one day and incapable of even basic functions, the next. This can lead to serious stress, angst and distress. And you may be the only one around for them to vent it on, so give them some leeway and help them find a way to accept the situation as well.

Sometimes, you may not be able to understand why the care recipient is behaving the way they are. For instance, a quote from an elderly gentleman who was looking after his ninety-plus-year-old mother is a good illustration. One day, he lamented, 'I look after her by myself, but she never has a nice word for me. My sister comes to visit her once in two months and they fawn over each other for the entire two days that she is around. Can you understand why?' Familiarity, boredom, a change in routine, associated memories, feelings of indebtedness . . . there are probably many issues at play here. Accept that their reaction to you may not be personal.

Most caregivers are an unappreciated lot. More often than not, the care recipient is unable to express their appreciation, and the others who are around tend to be more concerned about the care recipient than about the caregiver. This can make caregivers sometimes feel unwanted and unrecognized. It's nothing personal. That's the nature of the job. Accept it.

The main thing to realize is that acceptance does not mean there is no hope of change. The situation can be improved in multiple ways, and you will surely find many ways of making it happen. However, acceptance is a good starting point that allows you to look at the entire situation with a certain level of detachment necessary to make objective and sensible decisions without putting undue pressure on yourself.

After all, if you are going to be constantly stressed out, how will you look after your loved one and, more importantly, yourself?

Deciding on the way forward

The initial few days are likely to be full of decision-making, and which way you decide to go will depend heavily on various criteria, ranging from the trivial to the complex. The sex of the care recipient, your relationship with them, your religion, how orthodox your family is, size and constitution of your family, your financial status, the city/town/village you live in, the size and design of your house, the nature of the illness, the condition of the care recipient—all of these need to be considered. Some of the criteria that seem very important at first might diminish in significance as days go by and reality kicks in, but nevertheless, you will eventually have to address all of them.

It is important to iron out all the major issues at the very beginning itself, if possible, so that all the attention can rightly go to the process of caregiving. For the family, a combination of tact and plain-speak will be needed to arrive at any consensus. Of course, there may be contentious issues that may not be immediately resolvable, but taking cognizance of those issues is also important. This may seem like common sense, but given the emotional, physical and situational turmoil that is likely to prevail, conscious identification and addressal of pressing issues is a must.

The primary decision is usually about where the care recipient will live. It must be consensual that you and your family will be their primary caregivers. If there are siblings involved—or in even more contentious situations sometimes, when in-laws are involved—let them confirm that the care recipient is best served by staying with you, if not forever, at least for the time being. Once that is decided and out of the way, you can then figure out who will be involved in which aspect of the caregiving process and how the necessary activities may be divided.

The next three important aspects to consider are budget, internal support and external support. These are discussed in greater detail in the following sections.

Budgeting

Home healthcare is far from inexpensive. Depending on the nature of illness and the level of support required, it may cost anywhere from a few thousands to a few lakhs of rupees per month. As sensitive as money may be as a subject of discussion, it needs to be discussed as early as possible so that the required care can be given for as long as necessary.

Some of the most common expense categories are:

- *Hospitalization*: In most cases, hospitalization expenses constitute a major chunk of the overall expenses. If the care recipient has medical insurance coverage, some of this expense will be covered. However, more often than not, either there is no insurance (because the condition may not be covered for some reason or falls under the clause of some pre-existing condition) or the actual expenses far exceed the coverage.
- *Medicines and home visits*: Medication can cost anywhere between a few thousand rupees a month to tens of thousands a month depending on the nature of the illness. Doctor and nurse visits can also be quite expensive, with each doctor's visit costing between Rs 750 and Rs 2000, and a nurse visit costing between Rs 250 and Rs 1000.

- *Professional para-nursing assistance*: Sometimes, you may want to hire one or more part-time or full-time semi-qualified assistants to help with maintaining hygiene and to generally be of use around the care recipient. Such help can cost you anywhere from Rs 400 per shift per day per person to between Rs 10,000 and Rs 40,000 per month for round-the-clock care.

- *Equipment*: Most of the equipment will be one-time investments and, again, will largely depend on the needs of the care recipient. For Semi-Fowler and Fowler cots (which allow you to raise the head and foot of the bed), the prices start at around Rs 10,000 and can go as high as a few lakhs (if you want a multi-function ICU-ready bed). Additionally, if you need oxygen concentrators, pulse oximeters, nebulizers, suction apparatuses, blood pressure monitors, glucometers and so on, the costs obviously add up. Add wheelchairs, commode chairs, bathing stools and shower chairs, and you can be set back by quite a bit. Most Indian homes are notoriously senior-unfriendly, so you may want to set aside some money for modifications to make the home safer for everyone. More on this in Chapter 14 titled 'A Safe and Secure Environment for Elders'. Finally, if you need to set up a full ICU at home, the costs could start at Rs 7500 per day.

- *Diapers, underpads, wet wipes and more*: More than the one-time cost of equipment that you may have to buy, the cost of consumables is what takes people unawares. Month after month, the small costs add up and could set you back by anywhere between Rs 20,000 and Rs 50,000 a year.
- *Other expenses*: Apart from hospitalization charges and possibly medicines, most of the other expenses will not be covered under insurance, so budgeting and ensuring that you get the best deals from the beginning are of paramount importance.

Building yourself a support group

Most people who find themselves in your situation are pleasantly surprised when they realize that friends and family are more than happy to pitch in and help in the caregiving process as long as they are guided appropriately. More often than not, caregivers who feel they are not getting any support are those who fail to request for help from family and friends. In fact, it is quite common for the primary caregiver to be very reluctant to hand over charge of their loved one to somebody else, even for a little while. A mixture of guilt and lack of trust in the capability of others contributes to this behaviour, although caregivers themselves may not be aware of the actual reason for their reluctance. Watch out and don't fall into that trap.

The need to build yourself a support group cannot be stressed enough. On days when you are unwell, during periods when you are too stressed or when you need a break, it is always wonderful to have someone who knows what to do, to take over. So, enlist the support of your family members, extended family and friends, and get them to come and take care of your loved one while you are around so that they can get familiar with the routine and you gain confidence in their abilities. That way, when you really need someone to hold fort, you can quickly choose a qualified substitute you trust.

Apart from the main caregiving, there are many other tasks that need to be done, such as buying medicines and other required products, cooking a meal, sitting with the care recipient and talking or reading to them, hanging around and keeping an eye on the hired help, or just helping with the hundreds of other things that need to be done around the house. Enlist a wider group for these tasks. Most people are happy to extend a helping hand.

If there is a caregiver support group in your locality, either physical or online, join it and attend meetings. Though many don't realize it, interacting with people in similar situations and sharing your experiences can be therapeutic. Additionally, these meetings can also be informative and useful. If there isn't a caregiver support group in your area, maybe you could start one!

External service providers and what to expect

Doctors and nurses find it very difficult to make house calls. Many of those who do, often complete their full gruelling shifts at the hospitals and then begin their rounds of house calls—something which is understandably unsustainable. That is the ground reality. So, it is important to cultivate the good offices of a reliable doctor near your house so that in an emergency, they can be approached. If they are running a clinic, then you can also broach the subject of them hiring nurses and nursing assistants out to you if and when necessary.

Till recently, this was the only available option. However, over the last few years, a few home healthcare agencies have come up in India. These agencies provide doctors, nurses, physiotherapists and other qualified personnel to help you look after your ailing loved ones in the comfort of your home. Most major cities—and quite a few of the second-tier towns and cities—have one or more agencies that can help you. Some of these agencies are independent organizations while others may be part of a hospital group. They may be on the expensive side, but will make it all worth it by providing professional and dependable clinicians for your needs.

If you are hiring a nursing assistant—an unqualified or semi-qualified person to do some of the non-critical work for the care recipient, things are a little bit more complicated. Unlike nurses, physiotherapists and others who have properly equipped themselves with college education and work experience, most people who enter the nursing assistant profession are from the unskilled labour category. The reason why this complicates matters is that they are largely unqualified to be caregivers and would thus require inherent good nature and a lot of training from you to become effective caregivers.

You will find more details on hiring and managing external resources in Chapter 4 titled 'Managing Hired Help'.

Estate planning

Most Indians don't write wills, and this can create a lot of problems and ill will within the family. Try and get your care recipient to draft a will while they are of sound mind. This will pave the way for a non-contentious future.

Consult a lawyer and let the professionals handle this part.

3

Bedridden Elder Care

To just say that it is not easy to look after a bedridden elder, even with professional help, is a huge understatement. Truth be told, a whole army and then some are required to keep a terminally ill bedridden elder comfortable, if not happy.

We have dealt with several aspects that need to be taken into consideration at the beginning of the bedridden period in the previous chapter on Planning and Preparation. In this chapter, we will look at some of the continuing challenges faced by caregivers looking after the bedridden and share some of the collective wisdom gained by many such caregivers.

Resources involved

Space

A bedridden person at home can occupy a lot of space. In addition, if you decide to employ a 'stay-at-home', full-time attendant, then you will have one more person to share the house with. Consequently, the house becomes smaller and your privacy goes out of the window, and there arises a need to figure out what to do about this.

You could build an extension if you are living in an independent house or you could move to a larger house. Unfortunately, more often than not, you don't have these options, either because of money constraints, or because the process of moving to a new home along with a bedridden person is too daunting, or because you don't know how long the current state of affairs will continue.

You could, instead, prepare to make do with a house that has shrunk in size. Try and allocate one room exclusively to the bedridden person from the beginning, however difficult it may be. If possible, allocate a room with an attached bathroom for the ailing one. This will make sense in the long run. Of course, the attendant can stay in the same room, if needed. Here are a few compelling reasons why this is a good idea:

- You can maintain a higher level of hygiene in this room more easily.
- You can keep the lights on 24×7, if required, without affecting other people in the house.
- You will need to change diapers, feed, change the position of the bedridden elder and so on, at regular intervals, throughout the day and night. With a separate room, the care recipient gets the privacy they need and the rest of the household remains undisturbed.
- The elder may be noisy. Some might moan in their sleep, some might talk continuously during their wakeful hours, and some may even become violent—verbally and physically. Again, with a separate room, other members at home can be insulated from all this disturbance.
- You can keep the patient's medical records, medicines and medical equipment in one room. This way, all that you need for caregiving is available in one place, medicines don't get mixed up and the rest of the house doesn't start looking like a store displaying medical equipment.
- As you clean and disinfect, change diapers and give sponge baths, the room can begin to smell more and more like a hospital ward. With a separate room, at least the rest of the house can still feel like a normal home.

- You can air condition just that one room in the house.

Once you have a room allocated for the loved one, arrange the furniture in the room so you have ample space to move around. Refer to Chapter 14 titled 'A Safe and Secure Environment for Elders' for details. In addition, position the bed in such a way that there is enough space for a person to go around the bed. Moving the patient (especially when more than one person is required), providing physiotherapy and doctor's examinations—all become easier if this space is available.

Time

As a primary caregiver, a lot of your time will go towards looking after the ailing one and supervising the hired help. If you are employed or are a homemaker responsible for running the household, this is like having two or three full-time jobs at the same time. Don't make light of this and assume that you are up to it. The work, disrupted sleep and stress associated with this task can run you down well before you know it. And then there will have to be someone to look after you as well.

Do refer to the section on enlisting help in Chapter 2 titled 'Planning and Preparation'. Have others take on work on a routine basis so that the workload gets distributed evenly and you do not end up having to manage everything on your own.

Knowledge

In the beginning, unless you are a doctor or a trained nurse, you will be woefully unprepared and grossly unqualified for the task of caregiving. But you will learn. Most of the things you will learn are not taught as part of any course, so even though you start afresh, you are not particularly at a great disadvantage. The patient's room is your school, and soon you will be an expert. You just have to give it some time. During the initial days, things will appear daunting, but you will soon be up to it. Believe.

Read up on the condition that the patient is suffering from. Watch out for changes. You are in the best position to keep the ailing loved one comfortable. Symptoms can manifest differently for seniors and the bedridden, so have a good diagnostician and a geriatrician ready for consultation because sometimes, a regular doctor can misinterpret the patient's symptoms. As days go by, you will become an expert at identifying changes in the health

of the patient as well as the reasons for it. Consciously
seek that knowledge.

Fixing a routine

Any regular job requires a routine. A routine helps you
plan out your whole day and ensures that you don't miss
out on any of the activities to be carried out. Hospitals
operate like clockwork for that very reason, and with a
patient at home, your home is also, in many ways, like
a hospital.

If you are not already a person who works according
to a rigid timetable, it can be difficult to maintain
a fixed routine. However, with a little effort, you can
work towards a manageable routine that meets your
requirements as well as those of your family, the hired
caregivers and the patient.

There are a lot of aspects to caregiving and healthcare
that are naturally based on a routine. Medicines, for
example, are to be given at fixed times. Some, such as
medicines to control the thyroid, are usually taken first
thing in the morning. For the other medicines, the
doctor tells you which ones are to be taken before and
after meals, whether in the morning, afternoon, and/or
night. Similarly, diapers need to be changed regularly.
Depending on the brand of diaper, the outflow of urine,
and the medicines used (diuretics change the outflow

considerably), diapers may need to be changed two to four times a day.

Hired caregivers work in eight- to ten-hour shifts, usually starting at eight in the morning and eight in the evening.

Feeding is also done according to a schedule. The dietician would already have told you how many calories to give to the care recipient based on their needs. They would have also given you a diet chart to follow and told you how often to feed the patient.

There are also a few activities that are not conducive to scheduling, at least not initially. For example, a bedridden person's bowel movements may not be very regular. However, with proper diet control and the judicious use of laxatives, a proper routine can be established over time. It is important to do this as it makes life easier for everyone once a fixed routine is established. For example, once you ensure that toileting comes immediately before bathing, the level of hygiene of the patient will also improve dramatically.

Some events can destabilize your routine. Hired caregivers not showing up on time, or at all, illnesses and other unforeseen events can and routinely will throw your schedule out of whack. Some of these you will learn to predict and plan for as days go by, yet others will take you by surprise.

But with a routine fixed, the surprises will become less and less over time.

Managing bedsores

A bedsore, also known as a pressure ulcer or a decubitus ulcer, is a very painful condition that can affect people who are bedridden.

When bedridden people lie in the same position for prolonged periods (say three hours or more), some parts of their back get pinched or compressed between the bed and their bones. Consequently, the blood circulation to the skin cells in the pinched area gets disrupted. Due to this, the skin cells get deprived of oxygen and subsequently die. These dead cells form the nucleus of a bedsore. More and more cells die, pus forms and, if left untreated, this can turn into an excruciatingly painful ulcer.

Luckily, prevention is quite easy.

The first thing to do is to get an anti-decubitus mattress. Also known as an airbed or an alpha-bed, this device can go a long way in preventing bedsores from forming. Please note that the most common name used for this kind of mattress is 'airbed'. However, this is not just any air-inflatable mattress. This is a special type of mattress meant specifically for preventing bedsores.

There are multiple types of airbeds, but they all function in the same way. An airbed is made up of multiple pockets that are air-filled. There is an air pump attached to the airbed that is running all the time. The pump inflates and deflates alternate pockets in a slow cycle. So, if at time (T), one set of pockets is fully inflated and the alternate set is mostly deflated, over a period of one cycle (C), the fully inflated pockets will slowly deflate and the initially deflated pockets will slowly get inflated. At the end of the cycle, you will find that the originally full pockets are near-empty and the originally empty pockets are now full. This cycle continues 24×7. This ensures that no part of the body of the patient is under constant pressure, enabling every skin cell in the body to get its fair share of oxygen-rich blood.

Please note that the airbed is not a replacement for the existing mattress but is to be placed on top of the existing mattress. You can then cover it with bedsheets, bedcovers, underpads and whatever else you usually put on top of the mattress without affecting the functioning of the airbed.

Airbeds are very effective, and every bedridden patient should have one, whether they are at home or in the hospital. Many hospitals in India don't seem to understand the need for airbeds, so if your ailing loved one gets admitted to a hospital, kindly insist on having an airbed put in. If they don't do it, you should buy one and use it, as it is worth its weight in gold.

The second important aspect of bedsore prevention is hygiene. If the skin is in touch with urine and faecal matter for prolonged periods of time, for example, the chances of bedsores forming increase significantly. If you are using diapers, change them regularly. Refer to Chapter 13 titled 'Incontinence Management' for more details.

Finally, no matter what you do, sometimes a bedsore may still begin to form. This is where vigilance comes in. Every time you give the elder a bath, examine their skin closely. If you find any red spots, usually the size of a shirt button or smaller, take immediate action as this is the first sign of a bedsore. Ensure that you prevent weight from falling on that spot by, say, wedging a pillow strategically near that spot; keep the area dry and clean and then call the doctor. Follow the doctor's instructions to prevent the skin from breaking and the spot from turning into an ulcer.

Some people, including some doctors, think that using a waterbed can also prevent bedsores. This is not true.

Just to reiterate the importance of preventing bedsores, know that these pressure ulcers are very painful and take a long time to heal. As the bedridden person has only a few positions in which they can sleep, the same place can get injured repeatedly, allowing the wound no time to heal at all. In really bad cases, pus would need to be suctioned out on a regular basis.

Airbed, hygiene, vigilance. Repeat.

Anatomy of the bed

The bed for the bedridden usually consists of the following layers. The bottom-most layer is the mattress which is placed directly on the cot. An ideal mattress is a plastic or PVC-covered foam mattress of 3–4 inch thickness. This is a waterproof mattress as the PVC layer prevents any liquid from seeping into the foam inside. If the person is heavy, use a thicker mattress, otherwise a 3-inch-thick mattress should do. If you are using a Semi-Fowler or a Fowler cot, get a mattress that has folds in the right places. Over time, the foam inside will become compacted, so you may have to change the mattress every year or so.

On top of the mattress comes the airbed. This is usually made of PVC as well.

On top of the airbed comes the bedsheet. It can be as thick or thin as you see fit. Over this, you can put a disposable or washable underpad. The job of the underpad is to absorb any urine escaping from the diaper, thus preventing it from soiling the other layers below. That way, if there is an 'accident', the only work involved would be to change the underpad.

The patient can lie on top of all this. It can feel a little like the princess' bed in the fairytale *Princess and the Pea*. Without the pea, of course.

If you are not using an airbed, you can spread a rubber sheet below the bedsheet. This is mainly to ensure that the layers below the rubber sheet stay protected. Do not put the rubber sheet above the bedsheet as the patient's body should never be directly in contact with either the PVC or the plastic layers. Ideally, the patient should be on a cotton sheet or some good quality non-reactive acrylic sheet meant specifically for such a purpose.

On a daily basis or as needed, you will have to change the underpads. The bedsheet can be changed once every two or three days, unless it gets soiled. The rest of the layers can remain as they are.

Hygiene management

Hygiene is paramount. Maintaining a high level of hygiene can go a long way in preventing unnecessary infections and concomitant complications. Be it the care recipient, their room, the equipment, the caregivers or visitors, it is imperative that you aim for a level of hygiene that is better than what you find at a regular hospital. This process of maintaining cleanliness should become second nature to you. With respect to the care recipient, one of the primary focus areas when it comes to hygiene is diaper management. Diapers need to be changed regularly. In case of urine, the diaper needs to be changed before it gets totally saturated. In the case of faecal matter, the diaper would have to be changed at the earliest. You can read more about diapers in Chapter 13 titled 'Incontinence Management'. In there are sections specific to diapers with respect to the bedridden that you need to pay special attention to.

The care recipient's environment also needs to be dust- and mould-free. If they have a room of their own, ensure that it is maintained properly. This does not mean you have to be constantly dusting the place 24×7, but you will need to keep a regular schedule for sweeping, mopping and removal of cobwebs, especially if you have a frequent stream of outsiders visiting the elder one.

Needless to say, all the medical equipment will need to be kept sterilized and clean at all times. You will find details about maintaining medical equipment in Chapter 11 titled 'Common Medical Equipment'. In addition, it would also be ideal to keep a separate set of plates, glasses and utensils to be used exclusively for the care recipient. These could then be sterilized on a regular basis as well so as to guard against contamination and infection.

As already mentioned, hygiene is not restricted to the patient alone. The caregivers, family members and visitors must all come under the ambit of your vigilance.

We have dealt with the hygiene of the patient in many places in this chapter and book. In this section, let us pay attention to the hygiene of others within the ecosystem.

The first and foremost are the caregivers. The caregivers—family or hired—prepare the food, keep the room airy and clean, and are responsible for the maintenance of hygiene within the environment. They need to be clean too. All caregivers must wash their hands and feet as soon as they come home. They must wash their hands regularly, even if they are just moving about inside the house. They definitely need to wash their hands if they have given the patient a bath or have changed diapers. They also need to wash their hands before feeding or using any of the patient-care equipment. Other simple rules include keeping fingernails short, wearing a mask when near the patient and keeping away from the patient when they have an infection. Also important is to change into a fresh set of clothes as soon as they come home, especially if they have travelled by public transport or have been in close proximity to a lot of people.

The hired caregivers, especially the nursing assistants, may not have had any formal training on matters pertaining to hygiene. It is in your own best interests to teach them the importance and the necessity of maintaining hygiene.

These same rules apply to visitors also. Many of the visitors will be elderly relatives, people you have a lot of respect for. However, please do not hesitate to set the rules. After all, the patient is under your care and you are responsible for their health and comfort. So, get everyone to follow the same procedures that you all follow at home, when it comes to hygiene. And if any of them is ill, you are just going to have to ask them to visit some other time. If you find it very delicate to ask them to wash their hands and feet, have clear instructions printed on paper and paste them prominently on the door or wall. Additionally, you could also hand over a copy of these instructions to the visitors. You can tell them that these are the doctor's orders. You can find more on managing visitors in Chapter 9 titled 'Managing Visitors'.

Understanding medical equipment

Depending on the condition and needs of the patient, you may have to use a lot of different medical equipment as part of your caregiving duties. From BP monitors and glucometers, to nebulizers, oxygen concentrators and phlegm suction apparatuses, the list of products you may have to use can be long. Take your time and read up on how to use each of these machines. Ask your doctor or a qualified nurse to demonstrate the products to you.

Medical equipment for home healthcare use are usually designed to be easy to operate. Keeping the equipment clean and ready for use is by far the most difficult task, and most user manuals do not go into these aspects in great detail. If there are consumables involved such as filters and catheters, understand how often these need to be changed.

Also refer to Chapter 11 titled 'Common Medical Equipment' later in the book.

Importance of appearance

There was a young lady of Indian origin from the UK who had moved back to India to look after her ailing, elderly mother. Every day, she would give her mother a bath and dress her up in style. She would drape her in a nice saree with a matching blouse and adorn her with complementing jewellery. She would make sure that by 10 a.m. each morning, the old lady was attired beautifully and looked like she was ready to go out into town for a nice day of shopping. Only, they never went out anywhere, as the old lady was very sick and bedridden.

When asked why she did all the dressing up, she said that it was because when her mother had been healthy, mobile and independent, she had taken great pride in dressing well every day. It made her happy to look nice, and that was reason enough to keep that tradition going.

Most old people, however sick they may be and whether they are able to articulate it or not, would like to look nice. And when they look nice, they feel happy. While it may be more work for you, the experience of caregiving will also become more enriching because you are able to do something that makes the care recipient happy. For their sake, grooming is important. Grooming is important for another reason as well—when the care recipient looks presentable and happy, you will also feel happier. Try it and you will know. Finally, when visitors come, they won't say 'Oh! How nice she used to look! See what has happened to her now!' Instead, they would be happy to find the patient looking nice, and this will cheer them up too.

A happier and more cheerful sick room is better than a sickly-looking, depressing sick room any day!

Adaptive clothing

Dressing immobile people in regular clothes can be very tricky. While the above example is heart-warming, there is no denying the fact that putting on a blouse and saree on the old lady must have presented quite a challenge every day. Let alone a saree, putting on even a nightgown or a shirt can prove to be quite taxing, both for the caregiver and the care recipient.

However, dressing them up in a hospital gown is not always the right option. It may be okay during the initial few days when only the closest family members visit them. But seeing your loved one in a drab hospital gown, looking unkempt and sickly every day, is not good in the long run. Besides, these gowns never provide the proper cover or the dignity that you expect from regular clothes.

This is where adaptive clothing comes in. These are clothes made especially for the elderly and the disabled. They are designed in such a way that it makes putting them on and removing them easy, while at the same time, ensuring that they appear to be normal, well-designed dresses with cheerful colours and motifs.

There are clothes for people with different levels of mobility issues, including the partially mobile, the wheelchair-bound and those who are totally bedridden. Unfortunately, there are not too many options for these available in India, though a few companies of late have started manufacturing these in a small way.

Life will be easier all-round if you can get some of these adaptive dresses for your loved one. If you do, then as demand increases, eventually, more manufacturers may enter the fray and we all may start finding more options and better designs.

As a last option, if you cannot find such companies near you, you could always download designs from the Internet and get your local tailor to stitch them for you.

4

Managing Hired Help

At some point in time, you may want to hire people to help you look after your elder loved one. These could be qualified nurses in cases where the patient requires advanced support, or nursing assistants who can help with hygiene, feeding and other tasks to help the patient and assist the family caregiver.

Since the hired help is at your home for long periods of time, things can be a little more complicated than hiring personnel for your office, or hiring a cook or a maid for your home. Given the nature of their work, many times the line between professional and personal activities gets blurred, and this can lead to a lot of misunderstandings, which, if left unaddressed, can eventually result in you firing and hiring people on a regular basis.

In this chapter, you will find some suggestions on how to hire and manage the nurses and nursing assistants you may need, to help you in the caregiving process. These suggestions are consolidated here for easy reference, even though some of them may have been covered in other chapters.

Hiring right

Hiring nurses and other qualified people is usually not that difficult. You can approach your family doctor, a nearby hospital or a home healthcare agency and they will be able to find the right resources for you. Typically, since you will require qualified nurses and clinicians only for short periods of time, and that too only when there are complications, acquiring the services of experienced clinicians is usually not a very serious challenge, especially if you are living in a city with large hospitals and home healthcare agencies.

Hiring nursing assistants is a different matter altogether. Nursing assistants are people who are not necessarily qualified but can assist you in looking after the care recipient. They are usually needed for longer periods of time, maybe months or even years.

There are very few professional agencies that train nursing assistants for hire. If you can find a local agency that can provide you with the personnel, it is best to go with them as they will ensure a certain level of quality and predictability. If, on the other hand, you are unable to find an agency to help you hire one or more nursing assistants, either part-time or full-time, you will have to put in a lot of effort to find suitable people.

Since the people you eventually hire will be working closely with you inside your home, you need to think along conventional as well as unconventional lines. For example, as a first option, see if you can identify a relative or some other person from within your trusted network who needs some stability in their life and is willing to take on the role of a caregiver. A relative in need of a regular income as well as boarding and lodging would be an ideal candidate as it allows for a mutually beneficial arrangement. While they develop some sense of security in their life, you get a person who is a known entity, who possibly knows the elder one well and will be capable of doing the caregiving work with the kind of love and affection that would be too much to expect from a stranger.

As a second option, look for one of those few agencies that train nursing assistants for hire. Kerala, which is well known for the nurses they provide, is also becoming known for their nursing assistants. So, if you are in one of the southern states, you may want to look for agencies there. Some of the agencies ask you to visit them before they let you hire any of their people. This process is followed so that the agency is aware of the kind of people doing the hiring. Once they deem you to be a fit employer, they let you meet potential candidates and help you during the selection process. They have strict rules, but none of those rules come in the way of hiring and retaining a good, mild-mannered, well-adjusted, properly trained nursing assistant.

If that is also not an option for you, then you may have to approach your doctor, hospital or a local agency to recommend people to you. From them, expect no more than a list of people who are willing to do this work for a living. Through them, you would be very lucky to find a well-trained nursing assistant who understands the need for hygiene and is well-versed in the tasks involved in the caregiving process.

During the selection process, the first thing you need to assess in a nursing assistant is the level of kindness and gentleness they possess. If they are patient, even-tempered, gentle, have a decent sense of hygiene, can read and write even a bit and can use a phone properly, then they can probably be moulded into good caregivers.

Next, ensure that the applicant is healthy. You need someone who is infection-free as well as someone who is not likely to go on sick leave often. Additionally, some aspects of caregiving, such as moving the patient, require a fair degree of strength. So a person who is healthy and fairly strong would be ideal.

You may also need to carefully consider the gender of the attendant you want to hire. For example, if the care recipient is male and well-built or difficult to handle, you may want to consider hiring a male attendant as they are usually better equipped to handle situations demanding physical strength. On the other hand, if you are a woman and alone at home for long periods of time with just the care recipient for company, you may want to take into consideration other factors, including your personal safety, before taking a decision. You are the best judge.

Remember, apart from training them in the various activities involved in the caregiving process itself, you will have to spend time educating them on various other aspects, including punctuality and timeliness, hygiene and cleanliness, and the need to communicate early if they want leave or time off so that you can plan out your alternatives. Therefore, choose a person who is willing to learn.

After you have shortlisted a person, check on their family background. Do a reference check. Get the police to give you security clearance if such a facility is available in your area. Visit their place of residence and meet the rest of their family, if possible, and collect photocopies of their ration card, Aadhar card or any other formally recognized identity-related documents. Make sure that they know you are serious about security. If you have any doubts at this stage about their trustworthiness, move on and find another person.

At the end, if you are convinced that they will be able to discharge their duties well and can live comfortably on the salary you plan to give them, hire them.

Regarding salaries, one of the reasons why there are disproportionately more women than men willing to work as nursing assistants has to do with the prevailing salary levels. A typical nursing assistant gets paid between Rs 10,000 and Rs 20,000 per shift per month. The lower end of the scale is not enough to run a household and is useful only if it is supplementary income. So, if this is a second income for the family, then the chances are that the person hired will continue to work for you. If not, then you must be prepared for them to leave you for a higher-paying job. If you find a good person, be ready to pay more money because having a dependable nursing assistant is worth more than the additional few thousand rupees you will need to shell out.

Getting the best out of your hired help

Handling nurses and nursing assistants at home is an art form. You will soon realize that you need to be their boss, colleague and HR department all rolled into one.

To get the best out of them, to begin with you need to understand a bit of their background, their aspirations, their constraints and how the industry works as a whole.

Here are some hard truths that we need to take cognizance of.

For a qualified nurse, home nursing holds very little attraction from a career standpoint. Unlike in a hospital environment, where they have the company of other nurses, multiple patients to keep them occupied and prospects of career advancement, in a home setup, all they have, to be very frank, is a dead-end job.

As for nursing assistants, especially in the case of women, many of them typically come from broken homes. For example, they may be widowed with children to look after or have a drunken husband to manage. Also, in all probability, they have a household to run aside from working a full shift at your place.

Now, consider the constraints of their work environment. One, in many of the houses where they work, hired help is hired help. Family members don't socialize or have long conversations with them. This means that the nurses/assistants don't have anyone to talk to, except over the phone. Two, even a patient requiring round-the-clock care does not require constant attention. Thus, they have a lot of time on their hands with nothing to do.

Finally, even if they do a phenomenal job, it is not going to lead to a promotion or even a raise.

Under the circumstances, it should not come as a surprise if they seem to be on the phone for long periods of time or are not cheerful throughout the day. As you can surmise, given the above reasons, providing them an environment that will bring the best out of them is not easy. However, with a judicious combination of a firm hand and a friendly shoulder, you can have an efficient team at your service.

Here are a few dos and don'ts to help you keep your caregiving workforce happy and productive:

- Clearly outline their responsibilities. Fix working hours and break timings, and ensure that they are adhered to.
- Ensure that they only work one shift per day. Also make sure they have one day off per week.
- Get into a written agreement with them on salaries and bonuses.
- Have a clear leave policy. For example, define how many days they can take off in a month. Define how much notice they need to give in case they want to apply for leave and have a well-defined process for leave application and sanction, just the way you would expect at a regular office.
- Budget for unplanned bonuses. A festival bonus or a gift of appreciation at an appropriate time can keep them in good spirits and committed to your service. If you have a separate budget allocation

for social causes/charity, see if some of that can go towards making their life better. You could consider contributing towards their children's education or use the amount to help them repay outstanding loans that they may have taken at exorbitant interest rates in the past.

- Ensure that they are in good health and are well looked-after by you. After all, it is in your best interests to help them remain fit for duty. If you need a person on night duty who needs to be awake all the time—in cases where the care recipient needs constant monitoring and support—ensure that the person gets to rest during the day. Most people who go back to their home after night duty don't have the option of resting well during the day. Usually, they have their own work to do during the day. In the case of women, they may have to cook and do other housework at home. Besides, day times are generally noisy and are not ideal for undisturbed sleep. These are some things you need to factor in. Of course, if you have space at home, you could consider hiring live-in help. Though this means having another person living in your house, the advantages can more than make up for whatever loss of privacy and space you may experience. For one, there will be no unexpected no-shows. Also, you can ensure that they get their rest during the day and are fresh for duty in the evening. Finally, if cared for well, they will extend their help beyond their call of duty in an emergency, willingly and cheerfully.

- Show some leniency if they are on the phone talking to someone during working hours, provided they are not neglecting their duty. Obviously, you may have to intervene if it exceeds what you consider to be acceptable levels.

- Keep all interactions with them civil and cordial.

- Choose furniture for the caregiver carefully. If they only need to be in the room and can sleep lightly until called by the care recipient, then you could consider providing them a comfortable bed. If they are required to be vigilant most of the time, then a comfortable chair is a good option. If they need to be on their toes all the time, then a straight-backed chair may be in order. The key is to ensure that the caregiver is as comfortable as possible while being able to do their duty properly.

- If the care recipient is being unreasonable or uncooperative, be supportive of the hired help. You could do this by taking them aside and letting them know that you are aware of what is happening and that you will either be taking corrective measures, or, if that is not possible, that you are sympathetic.

- Do not give them any work that is not part of their job description. Even if they have a lot of free time, do not ask them to cook, make tea, massage your legs or anything else that they have not signed up for. If they volunteer and you accept, understand that you may also have to loosen some of the rules on your side.
- Do not reprimand them in front of others. If you need to correct them, do it one-on-one.
- Do not leave valuables and money lying around. This way, the hired help is not unnecessarily tempted. Also, if something does get misplaced or lost, do not jump the gun and suspect the hired help immediately. You risk doing grave injustice to a hard-working, innocent person.
- If possible, set up a CCTV camera and ensure that everyone knows that the room is under constant monitoring. This will ensure that no one gets any wrong ideas, while also encouraging everyone to be at their best at all times.

In addition to being efficient and reliable, if you need them to be kind and caring too, it is important to remember two other factors: one, how you treat them will determine how they treat the care recipient. So, if you are kind to them, in turn they will be kind to the care recipient, even when you are not around; two, how you treat the care recipient will be their cue on how to treat the care recipient. If you are unfailingly gentle and loving to your loved one, the hired help will also automatically follow suit.

5

Managing Medication

An important aspect of caregiving is the administration of correct medicines at the appropriate times. While most doctors' instructions are fairly straightforward and clear, lay people still end up making simple mistakes. This chapter provides a few pointers to help you avoid these basic errors.

Medicines, as you know, can be given in multiple ways. Some of the usual ways in which medication is administered include tablets and pills—taken orally or as suppositories, syrups, drops (eyes, ears, nasal), via drips and injections (intravenous, intramuscular and subcutaneous), through patches, and using nebulizers. In addition, there are topical creams and lotions for skin infections and pain relief. If you do not have a background in medicine, you may not be familiar with some of these terms.

Oral tablets are the most common way of administering medicine. They are usually sugar-coated and hard, or in the form of capsules usually made of gelatin. These need to be swallowed by the patient. In cases where the patient is unable to swallow, most often the tablet is powdered and administered along with solid or liquid food. This method, however, is not always appropriate. Some tablets are made to be slow-release tablets (that is, they dissolve slowly and release the medicine in small quantities over an extended period of time). **These should never be powdered and administered**. If there is a slow-release medicine to be administered and your loved one is unable to swallow it, ask the doctor how to administer the medication and they will be able to guide you appropriately.

A suppository is a tablet that is administered through the rectum, the vagina or the urethra. Most commonly, some types of laxatives are inserted into the anus where they dissolve and get absorbed by the body. Such tablets are clearly marked, and the doctor will usually indicate the way they need to be administered.

If the doctor has prescribed a syrup and if the care recipient is diabetic, check if there is a sugarless alternative as most syrups are flavoured and sweetened to mask the taste of the actual medicine. Also check whether the syrup is to be diluted first or not. As with any other newly prescribed medicine, read the instructions carefully before administering.

Drops are medicine in liquid form administered directly into the eyes, ears or nose. The bottles are usually shaped appropriately. Care is to be taken to ensure that the nozzle remains covered when not in use and is clean. Especially in the case of eye drops, ensure that the nozzle does not touch the eye of the patient. Most of these medicines, once opened, expire fairly quickly. Always check their 'use by' date. This is, of course, true for all medicines.

Saline, dextrose and blood (usually not at home) are the liquids administered through drips. In the case of saline and dextrose, match the strength against the prescription. Usually, a trained nurse or doctor will put the IV (intravenous) line into the body. This IV line can also be used to administer other drugs.

Injections can be intravenous (introduced directly into a vein/bloodstream), intramuscular (introduced into the muscle), or subcutaneous (injected just under the skin). Different medicines need to be injected differently, and you need to be aware of how each of the injections needs to be administered, even if the task is being done by a trained nurse.

Some medicines, especially lung-related ones, need to be administered in the form of a fine mist that can be easily breathed in. To create a fine mist with a liquid, a device called the nebulizer is used. You can read more about the nebulizer in Chapter 11 titled 'Common Medical Equipment'.

Topical creams and lotions are applied on the skin and are not meant to be ingested. Topical in this context means applied directly onto a part of the body.

As part of caregiving, you will come across these and many other medical terms. Take the time to familiarize yourself with the ones that are relevant to your situation. You can never tell when this knowledge could come in handy.

Prescriptions and administration of medicines

With the level of specialization prevalent in the medical field these days, it would not be surprising if you are dealing with multiple doctors for the treatment for your ailing loved one. While one prescription can be confusing, multiple ones can turn into a nightmare if careful attention is not paid to them.

A prescription tells you what medicines need to be administered when. Some may need to be taken first thing in the morning, while others may need to be taken before, along with or after food once or multiple times a day. All this will be specified by the doctor. The period for which the medication needs to be administered will also be specified.

When you have multiple prescriptions, it is best to have all of them together in one place and to make sure that each doctor has all the other prescriptions ready and available to peruse. That way, each doctor will know the details of all the medication the patient is taking and will be able to spot those that may not interact well with each other—this is called relative contraindication. From your side, ensure that you know what each medicine is being prescribed for. This will help you in cases where two doctors might be prescribing different medicines to treat the same issue.

Once a week, a responsible person should sit down and segregate the medicines based on the person's schedule, so that the person on duty does not have to go through all the prescriptions every time. This method definitely reduces the number of errors in administering the medication. Sometimes, there is more than one person taking medicines at home. It is important to keep one person's medication far away from that of the others', so that they don't get mixed up. Taking wrong medication can lead to serious consequences.

You also need to keep track of the possible contraindications and side effects of each of the medicines prescribed. Contraindications are the reasons why a particular medicine is not suitable for the patient. Usually, a doctor who knows the patient's case history well will not prescribe medicine that is not suitable. However, if you are going to a new doctor, it is better to share with them the details of all the other medicines the patient is currently taking as well as any allergies they might have (for example, to Penicillin, sulpha drugs and so on) in order to avoid complications. Notwithstanding all this, it is always prudent to check what is written on the box before starting any new course of medication. As always, go by the doctor's advice.

Side effects are undesirable secondary effects of the drug being taken to treat an illness. Some of the side effects may manifest in the patient under your care, and it is important to look out for them and inform the doctor immediately upon noticing them. However, this does not always mean you have to stop administering the drug. The doctor may prescribe other medicines to counteract the side effects or tell you to manage them appropriately. Sometimes, there is no other option but to suffer them. Again, do not go by what is printed on the medicine cover, as all possible side effects are listed there. For legal reasons, medicine companies tend to list all of them, and reading them all in one place can be scary. Also, do not share the list of potential side effects with the patient. Some people tend to worry about them unnecessarily.

Another safe practice is to start any new medicine on the morning of a working day (if possible). That way, if there are any adverse effects, you will be able to reach a hospital or your doctor quickly.

The period of efficacy of a drug can vary from drug to drug. This information is provided in the form of an expiry date printed on the medicine cover. At the time of purchase, ensure that the medicine has not already expired and is not likely to expire before it can be administered.

Please do note that a drug does not stop working the day it expires. So, if it is just a matter of a few days—especially for those drugs that have an effective period in years—they should still be good enough. If the drugs are older, however, it is best to consult the doctor, who will probably tell you that they should still be okay, but you should throw them away and buy fresh ones anyway, just to be on the safer side.

If the care recipient is in the habit of taking their own medication, it is important to ensure that they do not double-medicate themselves by mistake. After all, their memory may not be as good as before. To avoid confusion, you could get one of those pillboxes that are available in the market that have multiple slots for each day of week, marked 'morning', 'noon' and 'night'. You could then fill them up appropriately and ask the patient to take only those tablets that are in the slot corresponding to the day of the week and the time of day.

Finally, the same medicine may be sold under different brand names. Often, if the pharmacy does not have the brand prescribed by the doctor, the pharmacist may suggest an alternative brand. Do not go by the word of the pharmacist. Call the doctor and ask if the different brand suggested by the pharmacist is okay before administering it.

Generic medicines

A lot of medicines are quite expensive. One of the reasons why they are so expensive is that pharmaceutical companies have put in a lot of time, energy and money into research and development and they need to recoup that cost. They do this by pricing the medicines high. Also, in order to ensure that other companies don't just take their formula and make copies of their own, they patent their drugs.

However, these patents are valid only for a limited period of a few years. When a patent expires, other pharmaceutical companies can legally use the same formula to manufacture the same drug under a different name. Most often, as the actual content of the medicine is not that expensive, they can afford to price the medicine at a fraction of the cost of the original and still make a profit. These drugs, made using the original formula, are called generic drugs and they are just as effective as the original.

You can save a lot of money by choosing the generic equivalent of the brand-name drugs prescribed by the doctors. However, do not do so without an express go-ahead from your doctor. They should ensure that the generic drug is an exact match of the brand-named one in terms of composition, dosage and effect, and then agree to the alternative.

Generic drugs are not fake or spurious drugs, so if the doctor suggests that you could try some of the generic equivalents, do not think that they are suggesting something illegal. Generic drugs are completely legitimate and a boon to many patients.

Alternative medicine

Non-allopathic therapies such as Siddha, Ayurveda and other forms of treatment are usually clubbed under the term 'alternative medicine'. Kindly consult your primary doctor before you try any other form of medicine.

6

Managing Hospitalization

We all hope that we never have to go to a hospital. In an ideal world, our loved ones lead happy, active lives and when their time comes, they pass away peacefully in their sleep.

However, when you have a fairly old loved one at home, the odds are that a hospitalization event is never far away. If you and the elder one are both lucky, it may never happen, but in all probability, sooner or later, you may have to admit them to a hospital. It is always better to prepare yourself for this eventuality.

Hospitalization is a traumatic event for the patient as well as for all their near and dear ones. This is doubly true in India, where everything—from the availability of an ambulance to emergency readiness at the nearest hospital—is perpetually in doubt.

Preparation is the only way to combat many of the uncertainties in this process. Assume that a hospitalization event is around the corner. This will help you stay prepared in case of such an event.

Select the hospital

First, check with your loved one's doctor about their preferred hospital(s). If you have a choice, work out, along with the doctor, the best hospital for you, based on the quality of the medical facilities, its proximity to your home, the facilities they provide, your budgetary constraints and how comfortable your doctor is with that hospital. Get the list of ambulance services that cover your area and service the hospital you have chosen. Keep their numbers handy.

Advance preparation

Make a list of the various items you will require when the loved one is moved to the hospital. When hospitalization is imminent, use the list and prepare two bags—one for the patient and one for the attendant. Given below are indicative lists. You may want to make your own.

For the patient:

- Medical records
- Insurance details
- An airbed, if the hospital does not provide it
- Two or three sets of comfortable, loose-fitting clothes
- A sweater and some pairs of socks (since air-conditioned hospital rooms can get chilly)
- Two sets of your own pillowcases, sheets and blankets
- Two flasks, one for water and another for other beverages
- Plates, glasses, spoons and so on
- One or more airtight boxes to store medicines, biscuits, and so on
- A large wide-mouthed basket to hold all the boxes, bottles, flasks and other utensils
- Spectacles and their cases, dentures and associated containers (if they use these), hearing aids and additional batteries, if required
- Consumable supplies (diapers, underpads, non-sterile gloves). Some hospitals do not allow you to bring consumables from outside. Try and insist on these as the charges for these products at hospitals are usually much higher than their cost in the market.

For the attendant:

- List of contacts (doctors, friends and family)
- Two sets of clothes, a sweater and some pairs of socks
- A pillow, sheets and a blanket
- Phone, charger, other personal devices, headphones and earplugs
- Other reading material
- Medicines, spectacles, anything else that may be used on a daily basis
- Unused bathroom slippers
- Toiletries, including soaps, hand sanitizers, comb, toothbrush, toothpaste, talcum powder, makeup material
- A notepad and a pen/pencil
- A few tens of thousands in ready cash

Assign one or more people to manage the household in your absence if you are the one in charge of the home front. It could be a family member, a relative, a friend or even hired help. Brief them on their responsibilities and provide them with the necessary training well in advance so that the takeover can be seamless. This is especially important if food needs to be delivered to the hospital for the patient and the attendant.

It is not possible for one person to be the attendant for more than a day or two at a stretch. If the patient is in the ICU, there is usually no comfortable place available for the attendant to sit or have a lie-down. At best, they will have to make do with the uncomfortable chairs that are provided in the waiting areas. If the patient is moved to a room, there is usually some space for an attendant, but it is likely to be cramped and uncomfortable.

Therefore, to give every caregiver a chance to rest properly, you will need to have a roster with at least two people (ideally, three people doing eight-hour shifts) taking turns staying with the patient in the hospital. Identify and inform these people well in advance so that they are prepared to take on the attendant's role when the need arises. Additionally, you need people to ferry stuff (and people) between the home and the hospital as well as to go and meet doctors for various reasons. Again, assign people for these roles.

If the hospital does not provide an anti-decubitus mattress, keep a spare one with you for hospital use.

Finally, and most importantly, if the patient is covered under medical insurance, gain an understanding of the procedures to be followed. Ask the insurance provider to describe the process in detail. Get to know what the insurance covers and what it does not. Find out what the coverage limit is. Understand what it will take to get a certain amount pre-approved. Some hospitals work seamlessly with certain insurance companies, whereas in other cases you may have to settle the hospital bills yourself at the time of discharge and then claim the amount back from the insurance company later on. Knowing what processes need to be followed at the hospital of your choice will go a long way in making the admission and discharge processes smooth.

Admission time

If an ambulance is being used to transfer the patient from home to the hospital, let one family member travel in the ambulance with the patient. In addition, have at least one other person follow the ambulance to the hospital. Get the contact details of the doctor at the hospital end before you reach there. If possible, call that doctor and inform them that you are on the way so that the hospital can be ready to receive the patient.

Once you reach the hospital, let one person continue to remain with the patient while another takes care of all the admission formalities. The person accompanying the patient should have all the details of the patient's condition, their complete medical records, the reason they are being hospitalized, the doctor-in-charge and details of any allergies the patient may have.

At the admission desk, if the patient has medical insurance, provide the hospital with all the details and ask them to contact the insurance agency for a pre-approval, if possible. Clearly state the name of the patient's doctor and inform them that you are there at the behest of that doctor. If the hospital requires you to deposit some money, be ready to do so. Arrange for the appropriate doctor to visit and attend to the patient at the earliest. If the doctor's preliminary visit is getting delayed, pressurize the establishment by following up until somebody responds. If that does not work, call your doctor and ask them to call their colleagues at the hospital to do the needful. Do not assume that the hospital is aware of the situation.

During the stay at the hospital

Staying at a hospital as an attendant is one of the most tiring tasks imaginable. For most people who have not experienced it before, it is difficult to figure out why, given that one does nothing but sit around and wait most of the time. However, it is truly an enervating task due to multiple reasons, ranging from the serious—anxiety about the loved one, stress due to seeing sick people all around and the recognition of the inevitability of death; to the mundane—lack of sleep, boredom and uncomfortable furniture.

To remain alert continuously during all hours of duty is indeed difficult. However, it is essential for the attendant to be so, especially during the early days of hospitalization, when the patient is likely to be in an unstable condition. As only a reasonably well-rested person can remain alert for hours together, there is a definite need for a roster of people to take turns at regular intervals. Ideally, a shift should not be longer than eight hours. Plan accordingly.

On the first day of hospitalization, get one family member to go around the hospital and get the lay of the land. Find out the location of the nearest pharmacy, the canteen, the X-ray room, other important and relevant departments, the nursing station associated with the room the patient is in, the waiting area, the most comfortable chairs, the visitors' elevator and the various entries into and exits out of the hospital. Explore the locality and identify the nearest places where one can find parking space easily at different times of the day. Identify nearby ATMs, cafes and restaurants for the times when you are sick of the canteen fare.

Get the details of the doctors who are going to do the rounds and the times of their visits. Ensure that an attendant is there at all those times, so that any questions that you may have can be answered. Finding these doctors after they have come and gone is an arduous exercise. Know who the doctor on duty is, especially during night times when only skeleton staff is present.

Understand hospital etiquette and be a model attendant. Some self-imposed rules to follow are:

- Speak softly.
- Use headphones when on the phone or while watching videos.
- Visit only during visiting hours. Turn people away outside of these hours.
- Limit the number of visitors to what is prescribed by the hospital at any given time.
- Ensure that the place around you is clean. Dispose of whatever garbage you produce yourself. The hospital cleaning crew is there to look after the needs of the hospital and not to clean up after you.
- Don't wear strong perfumes.
- Avoid consuming food in the patient's room.
- Have a bath before you visit the hospital, so you don't carry any germs in.
- Do not visit the hospital if you are unwell, so that you do not to pass on any infection to the patients in the hospital.
- Wash your hands thoroughly with soap and water, or use a hand sanitizer as soon as you enter the patient's room and at the time of exit.
- Leave your footwear outside the patient's room. Keep a spare set to be used exclusively inside the room.
- Use only the elevators earmarked for visitors. If there is a board asking you to use the stairs, please do so.

Follow any and all other instructions given by the hospital.

- Assist the nursing and the nursing assistant staff in any way possible. Be nice to them and get in their good books, for they are your frontline support at the hospital. At the very least, keep out of their way so they can go about doing their work.

Sometimes, you may need some equipment that is not provided by the hospital. It is in your best interests to quietly provide them yourself. For example, if the commode is too low for the patient, get a toilet raiser fixed on the commode for the duration of the patient's stay. Similarly, as already mentioned, if an airbed is not provided, get one yourself (it will save the patient a lot of pain during the period of hospitalization and the subsequent days).

Finally, as soon as you get back home after your shift, no matter how tired you may be, have a bath and put your clothes for washing. You would have come into contact with a lot of disease-causing germs at the hospital and you don't want those lingering at home.

At the time of discharge

The time of discharge is one of mixed emotions. That the patient is getting discharged is, in all probability, an indicator that the loved one has made good progress and is ready to go home. At the same time, you know that challenging times are ahead, as these days a lot of the recovery is expected to happen at home post-discharge.

So, this section is divided into two portions—one dealing with what needs to be done at the hospital and the other dealing with preparing for a period of home healthcare.

At the hospital

The doctor usually gives you advance notice about an impending discharge. They may say something like, 'We will keep the patient under observation, and if everything is on track, we should be able to get them discharged within a couple of days.'

Then, if all goes well during the observation period, the doctor is likely to tell you to prepare for discharge, usually on the next day. Once you hear this, you need to take the necessary steps to put this into action. Go to the administrative desk and inform them that the doctor has given you the go-ahead for discharge on the next day, and ask what formalities need to be completed.

The process varies between hospitals, but the following are common activities that will need to be performed:

- Get the doctor to give a written discharge order.
- Get the bills finalized. This is usually a long-drawn-out process with the administration having to collate

information from multiple departments. If the hospital is a typical Indian hospital, this in itself can delay the actual discharge by a few hours to an entire day!

- Get a 'no dues' note from each of the departments, if required.
- Cross-check the bills.
- Coordinate with the insurance agency and make any other necessary payments. Sometimes, it is easier to settle the bills yourself and get them reimbursed by the insurance company at a later time.
- Arrange for return transport. If an ambulance is required, schedule it.
- Get the doctor to give a discharge summary that provides the current status of the patient and details about the care to be provided at home.
- If allowed by the hospital, tip the nurses, nursing assistants and other staff and share a few kind words with them.

At home

As soon as the doctor gives you the first indication of discharge, find out what you need back at home in order to provide the proper level of care for the recovering patient after discharge.

If you need any equipment such as hospital cots, oxygen cylinders and so on, make the necessary arrangements. You can decide between purchasing and renting, depending on the period for which they may be required.

You may also require hired help, in the form of experienced nurses or nursing assistants. If you have been nice to the hospital staff, they would be happy to suggest the right people or agencies to you. Alternatively, you can ask your doctor or friends who have been through this process or check the Internet for agencies providing these services in your area.

Clean the house and the room in which the patient is going to be put up. Read Chapter 2 titled 'Planning and Preparation' for more detailed information.

Living will and life support

Unfortunately, not every hospitalization episode ends in improved health. So, one must be prepared for all eventualities. Some of these could be:

- The patient passes away at the hospital
- The patient is beyond help and the doctor asks you to take the loved one home, so they can pass away in a more loving environment
- The patient's health deteriorates and they need to be put on life support

The third eventuality listed above is where a living will comes into the picture. A living will is a written and signed statement made by the patient when in sound mind, which describes the patient's desire regarding their future life-extending medical treatment in case of their inability to express informed consent.

On 9 March 2018, in the landmark judgment of Common Cause (A Regd. Society) vs. Union of India, the Supreme Court allowed people to make living wills, essentially giving them the right to choose what is termed as passive euthanasia.

What this exactly means is that anyone can choose to state that, if ever they find themselves in a condition where they need to be put on ventilator support but are not in a position to decide for themselves, they should not be kept alive using life-support system.

If your loved one has made a living will, please ensure that the same is conveyed to the doctor-in-charge and the hospital. Remember, it is easier to acquiesce to the patient's wishes and not put them under life support than to pull the plug later on.

7

Palliative Care and Beyond

There may come a time when there is nothing more that can be done to reverse, slow down or stop the progression of illness. At that stage, a patient is deemed to be terminally ill.

If the patient is suffering from significant pain and discomfort at this stage, the care that is given to the patient, where the focus is on alleviating pain and discomfort rather than cure, is called palliative care. Though, strictly speaking, palliative care can be given alongside curative treatment, for the purposes of this chapter, we will look at it in the context of end-of-life care.

The World Health Organization, in its factsheet titled 'Palliative Care', dated 5 August 2020, defines palliative care as 'an approach that improves the quality of life of patients and their families facing the problems associated with life-threatening illness, through the prevention and relief of suffering by means of early identification and impeccable assessment and treatment of pain and other problems, physical, psychosocial, and spiritual.'

In simpler terms, such care focuses on quality of life through the alleviation of physical pain and other distressing symptoms, through the use of painkillers or other treatments, and through counselling aimed at reducing emotional suffering both for the patient and the family members.

Unfortunately, in India, palliative care is still a fairly nascent discipline, and less than 1 per cent of patients get access to pain relief and other palliative care, according to the report titled 'Current status of palliative care in India' written by Mr Rajagopal, founder-chairman of Pallium.

Currently, there are less than 200 palliative care centres in operation across India. Many of them were started by individuals who were moved by the plight of the elderly and poor, suffering in dismal conditions during their last days. So, understandably, most of them are charity-run organizations focusing on providing relief to poor patients who have no support at all. Thankfully, having started thus and having gained experience, many of these centres have expanded their services to include sufferers who can afford to pay for these services as well.

Finding a palliative care centre

You can search the Internet for the nearest palliative centre in your city. The website of Pallium India provides a directory of service providers that can help you find the right resource.

Once you find a palliative care centre, you can fix an appointment and meet them with all the patient's records. Once they determine that palliative care is indicated, depending on the availability of facilities, they may be able to either move the patient to their premises or come to your home and provide the necessary care.

If, like many others in your position, you do not have access to a palliative care centre, then it is up to you to do the best that you can for the patient and find strength within and support without for yourself.

Improving quality of life

On this front, I am afraid the news isn't great. To begin with, the availability of opioids in India is strictly regulated and they can be extremely difficult to procure. If your elder one is suffering from pain, talk to your doctor and see what painkillers could be used to alleviate their pain and how you may be able to get the necessary permissions to procure and administer an opioid like morphine.

While getting access to painkillers may not be totally under your control, what is under some semblance of your control are the decisions regarding further medical intervention and surgical procedures. Sometimes, doctors do suggest medical procedures to alleviate suffering or to extend life. Meet with the family and discuss the pros and cons of these recommendations before making a decision. If the patient is able to participate in the discussions, get them involved and go by their decision. If they are incapable of participating or making a decision, then decide collectively, taking the entire family into confidence.

It is not an easy decision to make. Even the simplest of operations can lead to additional complications, pain and suffering. Ask yourself if the extension of life is meaningful for the patient. What would they do if they could decide? What would you want if you were in their position? Would the pain and suffering due to the new procedure be less than the pain and suffering that they are currently undergoing? Do they even have the strength and energy required to survive the operation? Many of these questions don't have right or wrong answers, and no doctor can give you definitive answers to some of these questions. Nevertheless, they are worth pondering over.

See if you can get a counsellor to join you in your discussions. If you and the patient are religious, it may be an option to approach your priest, *purohit*, *imam* or equivalent for guidance.

Whatever you finally decide, accept it completely and go with it wholeheartedly.

The inevitability of it all

All this suffering, the uncertainty and the lack of control can take a toll on you. However, you must remember that you are only human and there is only so much you can do. Ask yourself if you are currently doing as much as you can. If you are, then that is all you can do. Try not to go into hypothetical discussions. What-ifs are not very constructive at this stage. You cannot go back and change your decisions, nor can you be sure that any other path would have resulted in a better outcome.

Worry about what you can control and leave the rest to destiny. Death is inevitable, and you must reconcile with this fact at the earliest if you wish to continue to provide the best care that you can for your loved one. Also keep in mind that for most of the terminally ill and bedridden elders, death is the one thing that can permanently release them from their suffering.

Bereavement care

Grief at the loss of a loved one is a normal and natural response and should not be suppressed. In many countries, palliative care teams also have bereavement counsellors who work with family members for anywhere between a few months to over a year, helping them get over their loss. Unfortunately, you may not readily find any bereavement counsellors in India for you to lean on. If you can find one, please do use their services. Otherwise, you will have to rely on yourself, your family and friends, and maybe your religious guide to work your way through this phase.

One critical aspect you need to consciously take care of is the feeling of guilt that many primary family caregivers feel after the demise of the loved one. Every decision ever taken or not, and every act of commission and omission, can come back and haunt you. Doctors and healthcare workers have heard it all. Some examples of the game of second-guessing which goes hand-in-hand with guilt are given below:

'Four years ago, when my father said he felt dizzy, I didn't think it was serious. If only I had reacted immediately and taken him to our doctor, maybe he would have been alive today.'

'We gave my mother the best of care and she suffered for over seven years, completely immobile, and as nothing more than a vegetable. If we had been poorer and unable to afford such care, maybe she would not have had to suffer for so long.'

'When the doctor asked if my grandmother should be put on a ventilator, I panicked and said yes. If only

I had said no, she wouldn't have had to undergo the trauma of spending two months in the ICU.'

'I never said "I love you" enough times, maybe that is what broke her heart.'

As can be seen, there are no limits to our imagination when it comes to finding ways to feel guilty. However, it is time to move on. One chapter is over, and your life as a primary caregiver has come to an end. It is now time to rebuild your life.

If you are unable to shake your guilt even after considerable time has passed, approach a counsellor.

Rebuilding your life

After all is over, it is quite natural for you as a primary caregiver to feel lonely, depressed and bereft of purpose. In addition, much to your dismay, you may also feel a sense of relief. That is okay. For during the period of caregiving, you may have cut yourself off from all your contacts, stopped indulging in all your hobbies, suspended your career and, for all practical purposes, pressed the pause button on your own life. But now that your reason for doing that is no longer there, it is time to work on rebuilding your life.

It won't be easy for you to just shake everything off and start where you left off. But with a little bit of conscious effort, you can begin to start living your own life again.

Rest

You are, in all probability, seriously sleep-deprived. Rest and sleep are very restorative. Take time out to just relax and gain back some strength. Eat a balanced diet and eat well. Take a vacation. Get into a nice routine.

Reach out

Rebuild your social network. Reach out to people, even if it is just one call a day to someone you haven't spoken to in a long time. Invite a friend out for coffee or a meal together. Ask them to invite another mutual friend for the outing. Just get out of the house. You now have the time for it.

If you are looking to get back into the workforce, re-establish contact with your past colleagues and peers. Update your résumé. Refresh and update your skill set. Maybe you could use one of the many online learning platforms. Approach your old company or approach a placement agency. Give yourself time. Choose wisely.

Re-establish old routines

If you had been into regular exercising but had stopped in between, now is a good time to resume it. The positives of exercise go beyond just physical health.

The endorphins released during the process will make you feel better and help chase the gloom away.

If you had suspended your hobbies, it is now time to take them up again. Go for your singing classes or painting or whatever it is that you were doing before your life ground to a halt.

If you are one of those people who used to make it a point to go for a movie or a concert or dinner on a regular basis, go ahead and put it back on your calendar.

Get a move on. There is a bright and beautiful world out there!

8

Remote Caregiving

In today's world, it is not inconceivable that your immediate family is spread out across the world. This is great, in a way, for the elderly parents as it gives them an opportunity to travel and see the world without leaving the comfort and security of their trusted circle.

It does become a problem, however, when one of the elderly parents begins to need additional care due to health reasons. When this happens, most of the burden falls on the other parent who is also obviously quite aged and probably in need of help themselves, or the child living nearest to the parent. This person then becomes the primary caregiver, while each of the other members of the family either carry on as before or take on the supplementary role of a remote caregiver.

The role of a remote caregiver, that is, someone providing some degree of caregiving from far away, is a highly problematic one, both for the remote caregiver and for the primary caregiver. This is especially true in the Indian context, where a daughter-in-law often finds herself to be the primary caregiver. In such cases, remote caregiving can be fraught with tension, creating additional unnecessary problems that can lead to serious friction and even significant degradation in the quality of caregiving.

This chapter looks at remote caregiving from two different perspectives—one from the viewpoint of the primary caregiver and the other from the viewpoint of the remote caregiver.

For the primary caregiver

Remote caregivers are family members who, due to their circumstances, live far away from their elder loved ones and are thus unable to take on a significant role in the day-to-day activities of caregiving. This inability to look after their elder loved one at a critical time can be very frustrating and can lead to serious guilt issues. In order to compensate, many of them try to participate in the caregiving process in the only way they can—by giving well-meaning advice.

Unless the adviser is a trained nurse, a doctor or is in some other way qualified, their advice is largely useless and at best only reiterates what the primary caregiver already knows. This can be very annoying to you, the primary caregiver, especially at a time when you are already grappling with myriad issues that may be overwhelming you.

Desist from responding harshly. At the earliest opportunity, have an all-hands-on-deck family meeting. You could use a tool like Skype, Zoom, Google Hangouts or any of the many video conferencing tools that are available online for free. Set an agenda and run the show. The main purpose of this meeting would be to allay their fears, assuage their guilt and get them to provide you with help that has the potential to ease your burden. A constructive meeting at this point in time will go a long way in helping you manage remote caregivers in a way that is good for everyone.

Given below are a few suggestions for content and tone, but obviously you can do this in your own way. The important thing is to be sincere in whatever you do say.

Explain the current situation, health-wise

You could start by explaining the condition of the patient and convey any prognosis that the doctor may have shared with you. This will help everyone understand the gravity of the situation.

Take responsibility

You could convey to them that under the circumstances, you are thankful that the responsibility of being the primary caregiver has fallen on your shoulders and that, on behalf of everyone, you are ready to do the best that you can. This may not be totally true as none of us really want our elders to be unwell or have such responsibility thrust upon us suddenly, but you do need to say it and they do need to hear it. Besides, you are the primary caregiver, so saying this will allow it to sink in for you as well.

Be understanding and get them to be understanding

Tell them that you understand that if one of the others had been in your place, they would have done the same thing. This will help them believe that you are not grudging them their freedom. Also tell them that you are new to this and there is much to learn and it is overwhelming, but you hope to do the best that you can. This will send a clear message that instead of looking to criticize, they should be looking to help you constructively.

Enlist their support and gently set the boundaries

Tell them that you are going to reach out to them when you need help, but that you would be relying heavily on them for moral support, positivity and encouragement if and when you are feeling down. This will give them an idea of the best ways in which you feel they can support you.

Request for time

Inform them that while the role of a caregiver may be new to you, you are working towards streamlining everything. Request them to allow you some time to do so. Use this time to work out how you can utilize their services. Some or all of them could also contribute financially. You could also work out a roster so each of them can plan their visits so they do not overlap, allowing them to take turns being caregivers. At all costs, ensure that they don't all land up at the same time. This is counterproductive for multiple reasons. For one, they will all be happy to meet each other and it will end up becoming more of a vacation for them than a stint of caregiving to help you out. Two, you will be burdened with too many additional guests at the same time. Finally, with so many helping hands around to share the burden at the same time, they will not be able to appreciate the actual amount of work that goes into caregiving when it is just one person managing it all.

After this, you can throw the discussion open if you are confident that it will be constructive or ask them to come up with ways in which they can help however possible, from wherever they are. This will help you move them towards figuring out what *they* can do and away from what they think you should be doing.

Sometimes, because of cultural differences, for example, remote caregivers may not understand some of the additional intricacies involved in India. Say, if the nurse fails to show up one day without notice, you know it is something that is likely to happen from time to time and are reconciled to managing without help on those days. But a sibling in the US might jump up and down or go ballistic at the unprofessionalism displayed by the nurse and ask you to change the agency immediately. Little do they know that if you were to do that, you would run out of agencies pretty soon. Lend them a patient ear and calmly explain ground realities to them, emphasizing that you are ready to manage the situation. Help them understand and get them on your side. If they still don't understand, ignore them and move on.

Similarly, siblings and family living in developed countries may expect all the equipment and services to be of the quality that they have seen in the hospitals there. Explain using numbers, as in the costs for that level of quality versus what you have opted for and its sufficiency, and leave the decision of upgrading to the entire family.

Once you are settled in, have regular meetings, say, once a week. Discuss all issues. Keep the family informed and up-to-date. They will appreciate it and it will show in how they contribute to the caregiving exercise.

For the remote caregiver

As a remote caregiver, your primary job is not to provide care to the ailing one, but to provide support to the primary caregiver. If you take this to be your fundamental responsibility, you will be an amazing remote caregiver.

The primary caregiver's job is a truly thankless one in many ways. You have the power to change that and, in the process, contribute to the quality of caregiving received by your ailing family member.

Here are some suggestions on how you could contribute to the overall task of caregiving:

- Call and keep in touch with the primary caregiver on a regular basis.
- Call at a time that is convenient for the caregiver.
- Enquire about the well-being of the primary caregiver first and let the discussion dwell on their life, their challenges and thoughts, and their moods and experiences, before moving on to the condition of the ailing one.
- Couch any criticism in the form of suggestions and use gentle words.

- Plan trips to the patient's place as often as possible and go with the single goal of relieving the primary caregiver of some or all responsibilities while there. Do not treat this as a vacation or a supervisory mission.
- Send gifts to the primary caregiver once in a while. Just because! Don't wait for any special occasion.
- If you can, schedule vacation time for the primary caregiver.
- Share the financial burden with the primary caregiver.
- Take a keen interest in the health condition and the medical science behind its treatment. Understand what the doctors are attempting and stay involved in the progress of the ailing one, in medical terms. This will help everyone in avoiding conversations such as, 'Oh! I didn't know this'; 'If you had told me, I would have suggested . . .' and so on, which are both speculative and counterproductive.
- If there is more you can contribute without stepping on the primary caregiver's toes, by all means do so.

9

Managing Visitors

The importance of visitors

When you have a loved one ill at home, it is normal for friends and relatives to want to visit them and enquire about their health.

If, however, you have just returned from the hospital after getting your parent or grandparent discharged after a serious health issue, you might still be grappling with getting a hang of your role as a primary caregiver. At such a time, also having to manage visitors can be quite taxing and you may want to ask everyone to stay away, at least until you have organized yourself and your home properly.

Do this gently, as friends and family would also be worried about the elder one, and their enquiries and requests to visit are out of concern for the welfare of the loved one in question. Prepare a script and, if necessary, use the doctor as an excuse. Something along the lines of 'Thank you for your concern. We have just come back from the hospital and the doctor has given us strict orders not to allow visitors for a week or two. Once (s)he stabilizes, I will let you know and you can come and visit. My mother/father will definitely be happy to see you.' This will help in ensuring that the worried relatives and friends wait till you and your ailing loved one are ready to receive visitors.

Undeniably, visits from outsiders are important for everyone concerned and, in the long run, are to be encouraged under most circumstances. Visits from family members and friends also play a significant role in the recovery process.

Staying close to a loved one all day and being responsible for their health can take its toll, both physically and emotionally. Sometimes, to protect yourself, you may tend to behave more like a professional nurse/caregiver rather than the spouse/child/sibling that you are. This may, in turn, lead to a less loving and affectionate environment inside the sick room. Visitors help balance this out. They are affectionate towards the ailing one and to you, and that provides a safe environment for you to express your affection, too.

Visitors engender a sense of normalcy. Instead of family members constantly enquiring about the comfort of the patient, for a change the ailing one gets the opportunity to enquire about the health and well-being of their visitors. It provides the patient a chance to play the host once again and to ask the visitors questions such as, 'How are you?', 'How is everyone at home?', 'Have you had coffee?', or to invite them to stay for lunch, and so on. The outsiders' presence is required for such normal conversation to occur.

Visitors also bring news from the outside world. Being cooped up inside a room for prolonged periods with only the same few family members and professional help can get tiring. Visitors are like a breath of fresh air. They bring news from the big world outside and offer a chance to gossip, to catch up and to have a laugh (or even a cathartic cry). Visitors alleviate boredom and inject variety into the life of the imprisoned elder.

At the end of the day, if you weigh the pros and cons of having visitors, the advantages far outweigh the inconveniences.

Preparing visitors for the first meeting

Indian visitors are a strange lot. You can never tell what they might do. So, it is important that you prepare yourself, the ailing one and the visitors before their first visit.

Prepare yourself to be vigilant and yet be ready to give the visitors some space. As a primary caregiver, you will naturally be very protective of the ailing member and that is not wrong. However, if you come across as someone who is possessive or 'helicoptering', it may create unnecessary tension all around. Having said that, one cannot overstate the importance of being vigilant. The best thing to do is to keep your eyes peeled for potential problems while appearing nonchalant. Think of yourself as a superspy!

To give you an example of what a visitor might do, here is an incident related by a friend.

'I had just brought my mother home from the hospital and helped her get settled in at home. The poor dear was still in some pain and discomfort, what with the recent surgery, the stitches, and all the tubes going in and out of her body. There was the nasal feeding tube on one side, the catheter at the other end, and the IV line, and we were all pussyfooting around her and hoping not to trip on any of the dangling wires and tubes.

'The first visitor was my elderly aunt—my father's sister. She came bustling in, brushed me aside and declared that everything would be all right, now that she was there. And then, before I could realize what was happening, she put a sizable chunk of a Tirupati laddu in my mother's mouth!

My mother almost choked to death. Two people could have died that day as I was ready to strangle my aunt!'

This incident would be funny, if only it were not so scary. What is even scarier is that it is not such a rare thing. I am sure you can think of at least a handful of people who would behave just as unthinkingly. So, vigilance is important.

To help you start, here are some of the things to guard against when it comes to first-time visitors.

The insensitive one

The visitor will come in and immediately exclaim at how terrible your ailing loved one looks. Something to the effect of, 'Oh my God! How sprightly you were just a few days ago, and look what has happened to you!' Such insensitive and disparaging remarks can be quite damaging to the morale of the ailing person.

Before the visitor enters the room, prepare them for how the ailing one looks and insist on their making only positive and uplifting comments. You could say to them, 'Due to all the tubes and the drugs, he is looking quite unlike his usual, robust self. But don't worry, the doctors said he is going to be okay. Just be positive when you are with him.'

The melodramatic scene

This type of visitor will start wailing and lamenting loudly as soon as they enter the room. This will come as a shock to everyone around as, until a few seconds earlier, outside the room, the person would have appeared calm and collected.

Such emotionally high-strung visitors must be tutored carefully before being thrust upon the ailing one. Send them in with more sedate visitors. You can also tell them that the doctor has advised against loud noises and emotional scenes, as these can seriously affect the patient's health.

The religious one

As the episode described above illustrates, the religious-minded cannot even begin to comprehend that the sacred ash, *prasad* or any other religious offerings, though holy they may be, are not welcome near a sick person's bed. Catch such people early, collect the offering from them, and tell them you would keep it safely and include them in your prayers. Blame the doctor if they are difficult.

Boisterous behaviour

Some visitors act overly upbeat as a way of exuding positivity. They will announce that everything will be alright in a loud voice and go and sit on the patient's bed or generally behave like the proverbial bull in a china shop. Deal with them with a firm hand and ask them to keep their distance and their voice low so as not to disturb the patient.

The clueless

There will be some very irritating visitors who can't understand the condition of the patient. They will presume that the patient is deaf and a half-wit to boot. 'It's me. Do you know who I am? I am so-and-so, your such-and-such relative,' they will holler at the patient in a loud voice. They will keep repeating this while simultaneously entreating the patient to turn and look at them. They will do this even when the patient is asleep or clearly drugged and incapable of responding.

You can prevent this from happening by gently telling them that the patient is mentally sound (or not) and setting their expectations right regarding the response they might get from the patient before they meet them.

Most visitors are well-meaning, and if it is a new experience for them as well, they may not be geared to behave as expected. They may also be genuinely distraught on seeing a healthy loved one suddenly reduced to the state of an invalid, which can be a very unpleasant experience for many. Treat them as kindly as your frayed nerves and tolerance levels allow.

Maintaining a reasonably sterile environment

In many ways, a home environment can be a lot cleaner than the hospital. Some of the major threats, such as cross infections and superbugs, are practically non-existent in a home environment. In addition, unlike in an ICU environment where you are at the mercy of the hygiene sense of the nurse on duty, at home, you are the boss.

Keeping the patient's room clean and sterile is not easy. But with a disciplined household that is mindful of the needs relating to hygiene, this can be managed without too many difficulties.

The one thing that can upset your hygiene process is the presence of visitors. To begin with, quite obviously, they come from outside. That means they are likely to bring in dirt and grime from the outside environment. Additionally, they may have a cold, cough or other infections that they could potentially pass on to one of you. Finally, they may not be entirely aware of the hygiene requirements within your home.

So, it is necessary for you to educate them and get them to comply with some simple rules before you let them in to see your ailing loved one. You may find this a little intimidating at first, having to tell elders, educated people and even doctors in the family to take elementary precautions such as washing their hands and feet before entering the patient's room. But it needs to be done. If you are hesitant to tell them outright, you could print out the instructions, mark them as 'Doctor's Orders' and stick the bill on the outside of the door to the patient's room. Some suggested instructions are given below. Add/modify as you see fit.

- Are you currently suffering from a cold, cough or any other transmittable infection? If so, please visit when you are in good health.
- Leave your footwear outside.
- Leave your bags and belongings outside.
- Please wash your hands and feet with soap and water (scrub for a minimum of 20 seconds) before entering the room.
- Cover your nose and mouth with the mask provided.
- There is a bottle of hand sanitizer inside the room. Use liberally.
- Do not touch or hug the patient.
- Do not take outside food or religious offerings into the room.
- Do not touch or handle any of the equipment.
- Do not sit on the patient's bed. Use the visitors' chair instead.

Enlisting their help

Apart from the help that their mere presence provides, visitors can also be enlisted for more.

As you know, most visitors want to bring a gift when they come to visit a loved one. But what does one get for a recovering elder? Most visitors are in a dilemma. Would a book make sense? What if they are in no condition to read? What about some sweets or fruits? Is it safe to bring them outside food? A bouquet, perhaps? What if they have a pollen allergy?

As you can see, they are in quite a quandary.

However, you may be in a better position to suggest something that is useful. Again, it might seem awkward to do that, but it is really the best for everyone. You could request for some of the essentials you need—for example, some consumable that is not too expensive but tends to eat into your budget over time. For instance, you could tell them the brand, type and size of the diaper that the ailing one uses and ask them to get one or more packets. Or you could ask for gloves, masks, catheters, or even just a gift voucher from the pharmacy that you buy all this from.

If you don't want to do that or if you think the visitor may not be able to afford those things, you could always ask them to read to the elder or play Scrabble or some other board game if they both feel up to it, or just come more often, sit around and provide pleasant company.

Or you could just stretch out for some time and ask them to pamper you. You may ask them to fry some fritters, or ask about your well-being or maybe even massage your feet. How you can utilize their time is limited only by your imagination.

10

Taking Care of Yourself

No book on caregiving can be complete without one chapter dedicated to the well-being of the caregiver. A primary caregiver is the linchpin, the fulcrum and the mainstay around which all caregiving revolves. They form the nucleus around which all the others work and contribute to the health and comfort of the ailing one. If the primary caregiver is unwell or is not in the right frame of mind, things can go haywire very quickly.

This obvious fact, however, is not so apparent to most people. When there is a sick person attracting all the attention, somehow the needs of the others become not just insignificant, but are deemed practically non-existent. This is dangerous, both for the ailing one and for those who are taking care of them.

If you are the primary caregiver, it is important that you take care of all your needs too. And if you are not the primary caregiver, you need to pay special attention to the needs of the primary caregiver.

Understanding your role as a caregiver

As a primary caregiver, it is important to understand what your role is. You are the person on whose shoulders the task of ensuring care for an ailing elder has fallen. You are to do the best that you can, given the circumstances and the various constraints involved. Please note that this does not mean that you have to perform all the tasks involved as part of caregiving by yourself. Think of yourself as the project manager. It is your responsibility to ensure that the care recipient gets proper care, but you need not be the sole person performing all the caregiving activities.

In addition, be aware that the role of the caregiver does not completely define you, nor is taking care of the loved ailing one your only job. You continue to remain an individual entity, and it is not wrong to recognize and accept that you will continue to have your own needs, wants, hopes and ambitions. You may set aside some of these for a short period but you cannot make them disappear. Putting your own life entirely on hold is definitely detrimental to you and also to all others concerned.

Understand that the current situation is not your doing, nor are you solely responsible for every eventuality. Understand also that the physical and psychological demands of the job are going to be heavy and it is going to be your primary responsibility to ensure that these demands don't weigh you down totally, prevent you from doing your job as a caregiver, or stop you from having a reasonable quality of life for yourself.

In this chapter, we shall look at various ways in which you can take care of yourself.

Delegate

One way to make time for yourself is to delegate duties. Being a primary caregiver does not necessarily mean that you have to do everything yourself, but that you need to ensure that everything gets done. Allocate work and shifts to people in the household. Make different people responsible for different aspects of caregiving. Involve everyone. Make it a full family affair. Also, get everyone trained on all the aspects of caregiving. This provides you with a comfortable level of redundancy. So, if one member of the family is sick or otherwise engaged, another can seamlessly take on a different role.

Obviously, you have to take some of the tasks on as well, otherwise people will think you are just bossing everyone around.

Plan sleep times

One of the biggest challenges new family caregivers face is loss of sleep. This is especially true if there has been some hospital duty already, before the home caregiving began. Night duty is demanding. Depending on the needs of the patient, you may have to stay alert all the time, snooze with one eye open, or sleep lightly for extended periods of time. None of this can provide you with the kind of sleep you require. Even sleeping 'soundly' in the same room as the bedridden patient, either in hospital or at home, can prevent you from getting a good night's sleep. While on duty, your sleep is at best fitful, and there is no opportunity for the deep REM sleep that is required to feel fully refreshed. Sleep deprivation can lead to memory issues, mood changes, slower reflexes, reduced stamina and accidents. Long-term sleep deprivation can result in reduced immunity, high blood pressure, heart disease, depression, diabetes and a range of other serious health issues.

You know how much sleep you require, so ensure that you get it. You can compensate by sleeping more during the day and/or have people take turns doing night duty.

Balance caregiving and your career

If you have a job, things can get complicated. You may be able to take time off—a few days, a week or even a month, maybe—but beyond that, no institution would be willing to provide you leave of absence. So, you might either have to quit completely or find a way to manage both career and caregiving.

Now obviously, if you have a job, it is because you like what you are doing and/or you need the money. Either way, throwing it all away is almost never the right option unless you are about to retire anyway. So, more often than not, you have no choice at all. Accept that and explain to others who may need to understand the situation.

If you can, find a replacement primary caregiver. If that is not possible, get hired help. Try to cut down on your work hours, if possible. Explore all possible options before you give up on your career, for if you are like most people, your identity and your self-esteem are closely related to the work you are doing. Having to quit work because of somebody else can lead to depression, loss of self-respect, and sometimes even resentment towards the person who put you in that predicament.

Finally, if you have no other option but to quit, let it be solely your decision.

Make time for exercise

Your well-being is important. To keep well, you need to get regular exercise. A brisk morning walk, regular yoga or a workout in a gym are ways in which you can keep your body fit. Try and go out for the exercise. There is no fun in doing your exercises in the same room as the patient or even in some other room within the house. Let somebody else look after the patient while you are away.

Exercising not only helps you stay physically fit but also keeps you in a good mood. The endorphins released during exercise help alleviate depression, reduce stress and boost self-esteem.

Eat well

Now that you have a recovering elder at home, it is likely that you are preparing special meals conforming to their dietary requirements as set down by the doctor. In a small household, it is sometimes tempting to make more of the same for yourself, instead of cooking two different meals. This is not a good idea.

For better health, you need to have a balanced diet that is suitable for you. Make sure you cook and eat your usual food. Hire a cook if you must, but don't neglect your dietary needs. They are very different from the ailing person's.

Pay attention to your health

Do not neglect your health. Take your medicines on time and go for your regular medical check-ups. Caregiving involves a lot of physical work and this can lead to many issues, big and small. Do not ignore backaches, sprains, catches and even small, niggling problems, especially if they recur or are persistent. Do whatever is necessary to maintain your good health.

Keep in touch

As days go by, you will find yourself more and more cut-off from your friends. During the initial days of caregiving, when you are still grappling with your new responsibilities, you may not feel like going out with your friends. Your friends may call on you a couple of times and then, out of consideration, not disturb you further. The phone calls that replace face-to-face meetings would also dwindle soon as you will have not much to talk about other than your caregiving duties. Soon, you will feel cut-off from one of the most nourishing of relationships—close friendship.

This is bound to happen, but the remedy is quite straightforward. You have to realize what is happening and make time for your friends. If you already had some kind of routine with your friends (say, lunch on Wednesdays, kitty party on Thursdays, temple visits on Fridays), get back into that routine. If you don't have such a routine, maybe you could start one. Ask a friend to take the lead, or you could do the planning and scheduling yourself. If, for some reason, you are unable to leave the house, invite them over.

If they are good friends, they will find ways to meet you and spend time with you. But you have to make the first move because they need to know that they are not disturbing you.

Join a self-help group

Many cities have self-help groups for family caregivers. Most of them try and meet once a month or so and keep in touch more regularly online. Find one such group nearby and get involved. Not only will you find comfort among people in a situation similar to yours, but you will also find it useful in many other ways. You can learn from each other. Get tips and suggestions on things like where to buy products, which doctors are good, which ones do house visits and where to find good nursing assistance.

Once you have met one another and got to know each other reasonably well, you will realize that these meetings can be uplifting and energizing.

If you can't find a group nearby, then find one that's on a technology platform like WhatsApp or Telegram and join that. If even that is not available, maybe you could just start one in your area. It is sure to help you and a lot of other family caregivers.

Laugh, find happiness

Watching a loved one become bedridden, be it gradually or suddenly, can be a traumatic experience. That they are mortal becomes inescapably apparent, and that can leave you shaken. You may become sad and morose.

As days go by, you learn to accept this reality, but the sadness remains. After some more time, this becomes a habit. Visitors come. They are suitably sad and so are you. Essentially, you have forgotten what it is like to be happy.

Unfortunately, there is no upside to being sad. It only makes life harder for you, for those around you and for the care recipient. Soon, depression will set in, followed by stress and unnecessary guilt. This is neither required nor acceptable. If you find yourself in this situation, you need to shake yourself out of it.

The only way you can provide the best support to the loved one is when you are in the right frame of mind. So, tell yourself that it is not wrong to be happy, not a crime to laugh.

If you have a hobby, continue with it. If not, find one.

Give yourself a chance to be happy again. Go out and do what you used to enjoy. Watch a movie, attend a concert, go to a restaurant, do whatever it takes to shake off the melancholy.

Give yourself some 'me' time

Everyone requires some 'me' time—time that is exclusively yours to do whatever you want. Snack, meditate, read, or even snooze. It will help replenish your energy, give you peace of mind and slow the pace of things. You deserve it. Your care recipient deserves it. Plan it. Schedule it. Don't compromise.

Note to others

The job of a family caregiver for an ailing loved one is one of the toughest tasks to take on. There are no upsides and rarely any dramatic recovery on the part of the patient. This can be very taxing, both mentally and physically.

To add to that, given the situation, all the attention is understandably directed at the patient, and very little to the enormous adjustments the primary caregiver is making. Even though most primary caregivers don't knowingly resent this, many do end up feeling neglected and unappreciated.

To help them feel better, you need to give them some special attention. At every opportunity, enquire about their health, give them a hug, or tell them they are doing a great job and that they are so brave.

However, this is not sufficient. Understand that this is not a one-person job. As secondary caregivers, remember that it is also your responsibility to actively get involved in the caregiving process. You should be a part of the caregiving team. Do the tasks that are assigned to you. During emergencies, make sure you take on additional tasks without having to be asked.

As a mental exercise, imagine yourself as the primary caregiver and then list out the kind of support you would expect from the others. This will help you understand what you should do to be a thoughtful secondary caregiver.

Be there whenever the primary caregiver needs you.

11

Common Medical Equipment

With a bedridden patient around, your home will gradually take on the appearance of a hospital, thanks to the various home healthcare equipment that are required to keep the patient comfortable.

We are very fortunate to be living in an age where medical science has advanced sufficiently to allow us to provide even critical care in the safety and comfort of our homes. Today, there are companies that can set up an entire ICU at home, within a matter of hours. That too at a fraction of what it would cost for hospitalization. Having said that, in all probability, you may not need a fully equipped ICU at home. Listed below are some of the equipment used most often, that take care of a majority of the day-to-day home healthcare needs of the patient.

It is important that you, as the primary caregiver, as well as others in the household, learn to use and take care of this equipment. Most of the devices covered in this chapter are meant specifically for home use. However, some or all of them do require a certain amount of training from a qualified technician/doctor and should be used only as and when directed by a qualified professional. If some of the caregivers are illiterate, then train them well and supervise their work until you are confident that they know how to use the products.

Here are some common 'to-dos' for all the equipment you may have at home:

- To begin with, buy only good-quality products from well-known companies. Read the reviews and get recommendations from your family doctor.
- Check if there is a warranty associated with the product. If it is covered under warranty, keep the warranty card safely. Also understand what is covered under warranty. For example, for most airbeds available in the market, the warranty covers the air pump but not the mattress. Find out who to contact for warranty purposes—for some products, you may have to get in touch with the store where you bought the product, while for some others, you may have to contact the manufacturer or the importer directly. Please also note that some of the products require explicit online activation for the warranty to come into effect.

- Read the instruction manual thoroughly and understand how the product works.
- If it is a diagnostic instrument, learn how to interpret the results, and get instructions from the doctor on what to do if the results are outside of the normal range. You should know, for instance, what the acceptable range for the blood pressure of your care recipient is and at what value you need to get in touch with the doctor.
- Evaluate how time-critical a product is and ensure backup options. For example, if the nebulizer stops working suddenly, can you procure a replacement within an hour or so? If not, purchase a replacement and keep it ready.
- If the product requires power, ensure that a backup product or backup power source is available. Take the case of an oxygen concentrator. It needs to be available at a moment's notice. If you have power outages in your area, you must get a generator as backup or keep an oxygen cylinder ready. If a product runs on batteries, ensure that you always have spare batteries readily available.
- Learn how to clean the product and how to store it when not in use.
- Learn how to do basic maintenance of the product. Also find out the nearest place where it can be serviced or fixed when needed.

- Make a list of the consumables required and keep them ready. Some devices require catheters, for example. Keep a few in stock.
- Check how many times a consumable can be used or if it can be used repeatedly at all. Hospitals are stringent about disposing consumables after one use, but at home, you have the option of being a bit more flexible on the reuse front. Consult your doctor and go by their advice.

Airbed

The airbed is discussed in greater detail in Chapter 3 titled 'Bedridden Elderly Care'.

An airbed is used to prevent bedsores. It has two main components, an electrical air pump and an inflatable mattress. This device has to be powered 24×7.

An airbed can fail if the pump breaks down or if there is a puncture in the mattress. Usually, a puncture kit is provided along with the mattress and you can use that to fix the leak. Better still is to ensure that there are no sharp objects near the air mattress. If the pump fails, you can check if the fuse is blown. If there is some other problem, you will usually have to replace the pump as a whole.

Airbeds are available at all surgical stores. You do not need to keep a spare one ready as a person can do without it for a few hours, which should give you enough time to buy a new one, when required.

Nebulizer

A nebulizer is a battery-powered or electrical device that converts liquid medicine into a fine mist that can be easily breathed in. This method of administering medicine is mainly used for treating lung-related problems.

The main parts of a nebulizer are the motor-driven air compressor, a small, covered cup to hold the medicine and a mask, through which the medicine can be inhaled by the patient. Put the right amount of medicine into the covered cup after it is properly prepared. Place the mask that is connected by a tube to the container onto the patient's face so that the mouth and nose are covered fully. Turn on the compressor. You will see a fine mist forming and being inhaled by the patient. The process may take five to fifteen minutes.

Once done, wash the mask, the tube and the medicine container thoroughly, dry them and place them back in their container. Wash them again before the next use. It may not be possible to clean the tube thoroughly every time, so replace the tube once in a while.

If the nebulizer is used regularly and multiple times a day, you may want to keep a backup device readily available. Otherwise, you can buy one when the one in use breaks down.

Today, compact, portable devices are available in most pharmacies around the country. They are quite inexpensive and usually last for years.

BP monitor

Doctors and trained nurses use a sphygmomanometer and a stethoscope to measure blood pressure. The best thing to do is to learn how to use them as they give you the most accurate results.

However, not everyone wants to do this as it can be a little intimidating. A simpler option is to buy one of the battery-powered, single-button-operation BP monitors that are available in the market. These may not give you the most accurate readings, but once you have calibrated them (checked their results against those taken using a sphygmomanometer), you will have a reasonably good idea of how accurate your readings are and what the error margins are like. Most often, you don't need highly accurate readings, and as long as you know the readings are consistent and are not going off the charts, you should be fine. Besides, every time the doctor visits, they are likely to use the traditional devices instead of this electronic one, so you won't be going too far wrong for too long.

Blood pressure varies quite a lot during the course of the day. Time since food intake, activities done recently, level of stress, time since last medication and amount of sleep can all contribute to the variations in blood pressure.

To get the most accurate results, take the reading after about half an hour of inactivity on the part of the patient. The patient should be comfortably seated on a chair with their feet firmly on the ground and the arm resting on the armrest. Strap the arm cuff as instructed. The arm cuff should be at the same level as the heart and the marker on the cuff should be pointing towards the centre of the inside of your elbow joint. Please read your device's instructions carefully as they vary from brand to brand, before you take the reading. Repeat this after a few minutes. Take the average of the two and note it down along with the date and time at which it was taken. The doctor may also sometimes request you to take readings with the patient standing. If instructed, do so. If the patient is bedridden, you may take the reading with them in the lying-down position itself.

There are two numbers to note. The one on top is called the systolic pressure and the one at the bottom is the diastolic pressure. Systolic pressure is the pressure measured when the heart contracts and pushes the blood out while the diastolic pressure is the pressure measured when the heart is between beats. Understand from the doctor as to what the expected numbers should be for your particular patient. Do not go by standard charts. Call the doctor if the readings are consistently out of the range that the doctor has indicated.

For most reasonably stable patients, BP monitors are not critical devices. So, there is no need to have any spare devices. Keep spare batteries handy, though.

Phlegm suction apparatus

A phlegm suction apparatus is used to clear the throat of mucus when the patient is unable to cough it out. This device is also used when a patient has had a tracheostomy, to clear the trachea and lower airway of any mucus that the patient is unable to cough out.

Everyone produces mucus. In active people, this gets cleared automatically, and any excess can be hawked out quite easily. However, for many bedridden people, this mucus remains inside. Excess mucus, if not removed, can lead to breathing difficulties, pulmonary aspiration and other complications.

The apparatus usually has a canister that holds the mucus suctioned out, a motor that creates the suction and a suction tube that ends with a catheter which is inserted into the throat or the tracheostomy tube. Ideally, the catheter should be replaced every day. However, if you wish to use it for a longer period, it may be cleaned thoroughly and reused for a short period. Ask your doctor for their advice.

If you are inserting the catheter directly into the throat, ensure that the end of the catheter does not go beyond your field of vision. Make sure that it does not come into direct contact with the tongue, palate or the soft tissue in the mouth and throat as this can cause injuries.

If you are inserting the catheter into the tracheostomy tube, ensure that you put the catheter in only to the length of the tracheostomy tube and not beyond. You may need to ascertain the length of the tracheostomy tube before it is inserted. Again, check with the doctor.

You may find that some nurses move the catheter in and out of the throat as though they were trying to unclog a drain. That is not the right way to do it, and if you find a nurse or a doctor doing so, stop them immediately.

All the removable parts have to be cleaned thoroughly before every use. The canister is to be emptied every night or as soon as it is half-full. At the end of every session, suction distilled water for 30 seconds so that all the mucus is cleared from the tubes.

To clean all the removable parts (canister, canister lid, the tubing and the catheter), soak all of them in warm water with a mild detergent for half an hour and rinse thoroughly every night. For a more thorough cleaning (say, every three or four days), soak all the removable parts in a solution of three parts water and one part vinegar. Rinse the equipment and dry it with clean paper towels.

Phlegm suction machines come in electrical and manual versions. The manual version has a pedal that has to be operated to generate the suction. Where power supply is not dependable, go for a manual apparatus. In addition, if the patient is in need of suction at a moment's notice or very often, you may want to keep a spare machine at hand just in case the one you are using stops working for some reason.

Most devices come with a warranty of one year. This will usually cover only the suction motor.

Glucometer

A glucometer is a device used to measure blood glucose levels. Only an establishment with a drug license is allowed to sell glucometers and their associated strips. Most companies sell the glucometer cheap as most of their profit comes from the consumable strips that you need to buy in order to take measurements. So, check which strips are available in your area and their costs before you decide which brand to buy. There are two types of glucometers available: with code and without code. The coded ones require the corresponding coded strips. You will need to have a glucometer if the patient is diabetic.

To do the test, first wash the patient's hand thoroughly with soap and water and then dry it completely with a towel. Do not use an alcohol swab to clean the fingertip. Take a new strip and insert it into the meter. Check that the strip is not older than the 'use by' date. Use a new lancet (the small needle used to prick the finger) and prick the finger. It is least painful to prick the side of the finger's pad as the tip of the finger and the pad itself are more sensitive. Squeeze gently till a drop of blood forms on the pricked area. Make sure that the meter is on and ready before placing the end of the strip on the drop of blood. You should get the reading within a couple of seconds.

Wipe the blood off the finger with a cotton swab and wash the hand thoroughly. Dispose of the cotton, the needle used and the testing strip.

Please note that the glucometer measures capillary blood glucose and not venous blood glucose, so the results of your readings and those taken at a laboratory may vary.

Keep spare batteries handy.

Pulse oximeter

A pulse oximeter is a small non-invasive device that is used to monitor the blood oxygen saturation level. It is a compact matchbox-sized device that needs to be clipped on to a finger, earlobe or, rarely, the toe. Most devices are marked as SpO2 which denotes that the reading is that of the peripheral oxygen saturation. The readings are quite accurate and hence are used even in hospitals. These devices also measure the pulse rate, though these values may not be as reliable.

The device has a red and infrared light source on one side and a detector on the other. When a finger is placed between them, some of this light is absorbed by the oxygen carrying haemoglobin. The remaining light passes through the finger and is received by the detector. The amount of light received by the detector is then used to calculate the actual level of saturation.

To get the right reading, make sure the finger is clean and placed correctly between the light source and detector, fingernail on one side and the finger pad on the other. Since the device is like a clothesline clip, this is quite easy to do. A normal reading should be between 95 per cent and 100 per cent. Typically, if the reading goes below 93 per cent, additional oxygen may need to be given through a cylinder or concentrator. Go by the advice of the doctor.

If the readings take longer than usual to appear, rub the fingertip for a while and retry. Cold and clammy peripheries prevent the device from working correctly.

There are no moving parts in the device and hence it is quite robust. Typically, you may not require a spare device. You will, of course, need to keep extra batteries ready.

Oxygen cylinder

An oxygen cylinder contains pure oxygen in compressed or liquid form. It comes with a valve and, through a regulator and tube, is connected to a mask. In order to provide oxygen to a patient, you need to fasten the mask around the mouth and nose of the patient and, with the help of a spanner (key) which is usually provided, open the valve. You can then use the regulator to adjust the amount of oxygen being supplied to the patient. There is also an attached humidifier that needs to be filled with clean water. In case the user finds the mask uncomfortable, you may use nasal prongs instead.

The oxygen regulator will typically show the reading in litres per minute (LPM). Most cylinders can provide between 1 and 10 LPM. Obviously, the more difficulty there is in breathing, the more the supply of oxygen should be. The doctor will be able to guide you as to what the setting should be based on the condition of the patient and the current blood oxygen saturation levels.

Oxygen cylinders leak tiny amounts of oxygen even when not in use. So, it is important to check how much oxygen is left in the tank from time to time so that you have the oxygen readily available when you need it. The provider of the cylinder will usually tell you the capacity of the cylinder (in terms of litres) and how often it needs to be replaced (when not in use). Ask them about lead times and their working hours. Choose a provider who is close to your home and is ready to respond 24×7. Do a reference-check on the vendor to be sure that they are dependable.

Oxygen concentrator

A portable home oxygen concentrator is an electrically powered device that produces oxygen. It concentrates the ambient air to produce oxygen for home-based patients. A typical device is extremely low maintenance, requiring only regular filter changes, and will last anywhere from four to seven years depending on usage.

Small devices may provide up to 5 LPM and larger ones up to 10 LPM. Choose based on anticipated needs.

Since the device requires electricity to work, you need to have a stable power supply. The device may not work with a typical home inverter/UPS, so you may need to have a diesel generator on standby in case you have power outages in your area. Alternatively, you can keep an oxygen cylinder as backup.

Oxygen concentrators are available for purchase as well as on rent. If your need is short-term, renting would be the ideal option. However, if you need it for an extended period, buying would be the less expensive option in the long run. Many companies allow for payment to be made in instalments.

BiPAP/CPAP

BiPAP stands for Bilevel Positive Airway Pressure and CPAP stands for Continuous Positive Airway Pressure. These are forms of non-invasive ventilators used when a person finds breathing difficult.

We usually think that the air we breathe in expands our lungs when, in fact, it is the other way around. At the time of inhalation, the diaphragm muscles work to expand the lungs. This creates a partial vacuum in your lungs, making the air outside rush inside. Similarly, at the time of exhalation, the diaphragm muscles compress the lungs, forcing the air out. If the diaphragm muscles are weak or if the lungs are unable to expand for some other reason, air may have to be forced inside using one of these devices.

The CPAP pushes air into the airways at a single level of pressure. This makes it difficult for some people to exhale as they have to force air out of their lungs against the additional pressure exerted by the CPAP device. The BiPAP has two levels of pressure—one at the time of inhalation (higher) and one at the time of exhalation (lower)—making exhaling also easier. Some devices come with a humidifier to prevent the drying of the patient's mouth and windpipe.

These devices are recommended during the treatment of conditions such as Chronic Obstructive Pulmonary Disorder (COPD), obstructive sleep apnoea, pneumonia, asthma, post-operative breathing difficulty and certain neurological conditions that affect breathing.

If the condition is not alleviated by the use of a BiPAP or CPAP, you may have to go in for a ventilator with intubation or have a tracheostomy procedure done. Again, a doctor is the best judge.

Please note that the BiPAP/CPAP has to be calibrated for each patient. Also, there are different types of masks, and you may have to try them on before deciding on which one is the most suitable for your needs. The mask is a very important component and if it does not fit properly, there will be leaks, leading to insufficient pressure being provided.

The mask, the associated tubes and other removable parts have to be cleaned regularly. Water and mild detergent can be used for cleaning.

As these are powered by electricity, you will need to ensure a steady supply of power.

Compression stockings

Graduated compression stockings are used for many reasons, from improving blood circulation in the legs to problems such as edema, varicose veins and deep vein thrombosis. Heart and kidney diseases can also cause poor blood circulation which can lead to clotting of the blood inside the veins and consequently result in deep vein thrombosis and strokes.

If you have ever watered your garden with a garden hose, then you would have surely used your thumb to cover part of the mouth of the hose to force the water to go farther. Compression socks work in a similar fashion. They compress the veins in the legs (or hands) and force better circulation of blood from the legs towards the heart.

Compression stockings come in various materials, sizes and lengths. The lengths are usually marked as 'AD', 'AF' or 'AG', indicating whether they are calf-length (ending just below the knee), thigh-length, or groin-length. The doctor will guide you as to which length is indicated for the patient.

The size depends on the circumference of the patient's leg at various points. The size chart on the box will help you decide which is the right size using the circumference of the legs at the ankle, knee and/or thigh. Ideally, the measurement should be taken first thing in the morning, which is when there is least retention of fluid in the limbs. Make sure you buy the right size. If it is too loose, it will not provide the right compression, and if it is too tight, it will be extremely difficult to wear and can lead to other problems.

A compression stocking is not the easiest thing to wear and is even more difficult to put on for somebody else. Do not discontinue its use for this reason. There are products available that help put on and remove them as well as many techniques to make it easier to do so. YouTube, as always, is a good source of information. Note that the stockings lose their elasticity over time and become ineffective, so replace them at regular intervals.

Cannula

You have surely seen this, though you may not know its name. It is the thin tube that is inserted into the patient's vein, usually at the back of the hand, through which medicine is regularly injected directly into the patient's bloodstream. Hospitals use a cannula as it helps them dramatically reduce the number of places a patient needs to be pricked for administering injections.

The one on the hand is called a peripheral IV cannula and can be used for up to three or four days. The central IV cannula is usually placed near the neck directly into the jugular, subclavian or the femoral vein, and the midline IV cannula is placed where the veins are large, usually in the upper arm. The latter two can be used for longer periods.

Inform the doctor if there is redness, swelling or pain around the cannula.

12

Understanding Common
Medical Procedures

If you have a post-operative patient or an elderly person bedridden at home, apart from the illness-specific procedures and treatment, you are likely to have to deal with a few common medical procedures. These procedures are associated with breathing, food intake and excretion. Given below is a brief introduction to these procedures and associated post-operative and long-term care for the lay reader. Use this as a place to start. Your doctor is your best source of information.

Tracheostomy

A tracheostomy is done when the patient is unable to breathe normally for any number of reasons such as chronic lung disease or cancer in the neck area. The need for a ventilator for a prolonged period may also necessitate a tracheostomy. It is a regular procedure done under general anaesthesia. Briefly, a hole is made just under the Adam's apple, through the neck and into the trachea or the windpipe. This hole is called the stoma. The tracheostomy tube is inserted into this and fixed using a strap that goes around the neck.

Once the operation is complete, the patient will be able to breathe through this tube, bypassing the nose, mouth and throat. However, it could take the patient a few days to get used to breathing through the tube. Speech is also affected, and it may even be difficult for them to make any kind of sound during the initial days. Though the vocal cords (which are above the hole in the neck) are not damaged during the operation, the fact that air does not pass that way impedes speech. However, with practice, they may be able to regain their ability to speak. For some, closing the tube helps. There are special valves that can be fitted to the tube which allow the patient to breathe in through the tube and breathe out through the mouth and nose, which can dramatically improve their ability to speak.

Eating may also be difficult for some time, and usually a nasogastric tube is inserted till the wounds heal. Afterwards, you may need a speech therapist to help restore the strength in the muscles involved in swallowing.

If the patient is unable to breathe by themselves, then a ventilator can easily be attached to the tube.

As with any other operation, there are risks. Some of these specific to a tracheostomy include damage to the thyroid gland and lung collapse.

Post-operative care is very important. The tube and the area around the stoma need to be cleaned regularly and the skin kept free of any infection. Learn to maintain hygiene from a trained clinician. Doctors recommend cleaning the area around the stoma twice a day at least with a 50:50 solution of sterile water and hydrogen peroxide. Needless to say, any other equipment used, such as suction catheters and phlegm suction apparatus, should also be kept clean and sterile.

As always, consult the doctor at the first sign of infection or discomfort. Some of the signs to look for include bleeding, pain, redness or swelling at and around the stoma, difficulty in breathing, or a change in the position of the tracheostomy tube.

Ryles tube

A Ryles tube or a nasogastric tube is a small-bore, flexible, rubber, silicone or polyurethane tube used to feed patients who are unable to use their mouths for some reason. The tube is usually inserted through one of the nostrils all the way into the stomach or sometimes into the duodenum (called the nasoduodenal tube) if the doctor deems it necessary. The procedure is fairly painless and can be done by a trained clinician in about a minute or so.

The clinician will usually measure out the tube so they know how much needs to be inserted, lubricate the tip with a gel and then slowly insert it. Care is taken to ensure that it goes into the food pipe and not the airway. Once it is inserted fully, the clinician will check to confirm that it has gone into the stomach either by extracting some fluid and checking it, by blowing air through the tube with a syringe (to see if the stomach enlarges as proof), or by using an X-ray machine. While the patient may feel some discomfort during the process of insertion, once it is in place, the patient is unlikely to feel any pain or discomfort.

Once the tube is positioned correctly, it is fixed in place by fastening the portion coming out of the nose using tape. It is important that neither the patient nor anybody else pulls out the Ryles tube inadvertently.

Feeding can be done by using a graduated bag hung from an IV stand or using a large syringe as a funnel to pour liquid food through the tube. While you can prepare your own food, many doctors recommend powders which are complete meal replacements. These are easy to mix, do not form lumps and meet the dietary requirements of most patients. Flush the tube with

30 ml of water after every meal or once in four hours, whichever is more frequent.

Ryles tubes are usually used only for short durations of up to two weeks, but they can be used for longer periods also.

Needless to say, cleanliness is of paramount importance.

Percutaneous Endoscopic Gastrostomy (PEG)

Usually referred to as PEG, this is a procedure by which a feeding tube is inserted into the stomach directly through the abdominal wall. This allows fluids, medication and food to be introduced directly into the stomach, bypassing the mouth and the esophagus.

The procedure is a fairly straightforward one and is often done under local anaesthesia. If all goes well, the patient can be back home even on the very same day.

Briefly, the doctor inserts an endoscope through the mouth into the stomach. The endoscope has a light which is then shined outwards. This helps the doctor identify the exact location and position of the stomach. Using this as a reference, the doctor then makes a small incision in the abdominal wall and the stomach wall, and then inserts a small tube and fixes it in position. The tube can be in place from a few months to even up to a few years. If it gets clogged or dislodged, it can be replaced in the same place or at another location. Removal is usually done endoscopically. In simple terms, the outer portion of the tube is cut and the rest of the tube is pushed into the stomach and then, using an endoscopic snare, it is removed through the mouth. The PEG site then is left to heal by itself.

A PEG is a good alternative to long-term Ryles tube usage. You should consider this option if normal and nasogastric feeding are not possible. This could happen in the case of a stroke, certain neurological conditions, or tumours in the head, neck and esophageal areas. Like in most procedures, there can be complications, though by and large this is a straightforward procedure and has long-term benefits over nasogastric tubes.

Many hospitals in India are capable of performing this procedure. In fact, if you broach the subject, most doctors oblige with alacrity. Get a second and a third opinion before deciding on this procedure.

It is important to confirm four things: one, whether it is absolutely essential; two, that there are no contraindications; three, that this will be an improvement over the current situation and effective for a considerable period of time; and finally, that the patient will be able to take the trauma of hospitalization and the procedure, simple though it might be.

Once the operation is done, ensure that you keep the PEG site clean and keep a keen eye out for any infection or discolouration in that area.

Urinary catheters

Urinary catheterization is the process of placing a catheter up the urethra into the bladder to enable draining of the bladder. The catheter is a thin tube made of latex, polyurethane or silicone.

You will see the use of a urinary catheter usually after a surgery. Most often, the catheter used is of a type called Foley's catheter. This has a small inflatable balloon at the end. The person who performs this procedure, usually a trained nurse, will slowly insert the catheter into the urethra until its tip reaches the bladder. Then they will inject saline water so the balloon at the tip of the catheter gets inflated and is thus held in place. There are different catheters for men and women, the main difference being the size of the balloon at the end.

Most often, the catheter ends in a collection bag that is hung on a hook at the bottom of the bed. Do not leave this bag on the floor, as it can lead to bacterial infection. This bag collects the urine and has to be emptied from time to time. These bags also usually have calibration markings on the outside that allow you to measure the outflow. If the quantity collected is too low or the flow stops completely, inform the doctor immediately.

When the patient becomes mobile, this bag may be replaced by a smaller bag that can be strapped to the leg. This makes the catheter less conspicuous, thus allowing the patient to walk around without feeling self-conscious. There is also another kind of bag that can be strapped to the belly region.

Though people can be trained to do self-catheterization, this is mostly applicable for younger people who need it. For elders, it is always better for a trained clinician to perform the procedure.

Urinary catheterization is not without its problems. Complications include urinary tract infection, blood infection, urethral damage and blood in urine. To avoid these problems, additional care is required. Some of the things you need to do are:

- Keep the tubing out of the way so that no one trips on it or pulls it inadvertently as this can cause serious damage.
- Clean the tip of the urethra (the point where the catheter exits the body) on a regular basis. The catheter also needs to be cleaned regularly.
- Disconnect and connect the drainage bag using clean hands.
- Do not leave the bag lying around.
- Make sure only a trained nurse does the insertion and removal of the catheter. An untrained person may damage the urethra, which can lead to additional complications.

- Have a nurse do a bladder washout at least once every ten days. During this process, a sterile liquid is introduced into the bladder via the catheter and then drained. This helps in removing any blood clots in the bladder and catheter and ensures better draining of the bladder.

For men, there is one more type of catheter called a condom catheter. This is a non-invasive type and works as the name suggests. This catheter looks like a modified condom, a sheath with a tube at the end that can be rolled on to the penis. They come in different sizes, so you need to refer to the sizing chart on the product to find the right one for the patient. This type of external catheter is used only in the case of male urinary incontinence. This does not help if the patient is unable to empty the bladder.

Colostomy

When there are problems with the lower intestinal tract or the anus, passing stools the regular way may become difficult or even impossible. Under such circumstances, doctors perform a procedure called a colostomy.

This involves making an incision in the abdominal wall and bringing the end of the large intestine out through the hole to connect it to a bag that can collect the faeces. This helps in bypassing the parts of the large intestines or the anal region which may be the source of the problem.

A colostomy is a major surgery and carries associated risks. If it is a regular surgery, the incision made is large. If it is a laparoscopic surgery, several smaller incisions will be made. A ring is then fixed to the abdominal wall. Then the large intestine is cut at the appropriate place and brought out through the ring and fixed with sutures. The ring may be the permanent kind or a temporary one. Some of the risks include hernia, internal bleeding, damage to other organs, infection and problems relating to scar tissue. After the surgery, there will be diet restrictions and these will need to be adhered to strictly.

Get a trained clinician to teach you the process of changing the colostomy pouch and maintaining the area around the stoma clean. Watch them do it a few times, and then do it a few times yourself under their direct supervision. You may have to do this once or twice a day. If it is not done properly, it can lead to a lot of problems.

The pouch may be a one-piece system or may come in two parts. In the two-piece system, the skin barrier comes separately. The skin barrier sticks to the skin around the stoma and provides a way for the rest of the pouch to be attached to it. Choose a pouch that is the right size for the patient.

Depending on the type of pouch, you may have to change it every time there is a bowel movement or once every few hours. Check with the doctor and the manufacturer of the pouch.

During changing, remove the pouch carefully to ensure that there is no spillage. Remove the skin barrier if required. Clean the area around the stoma thoroughly. Check that there is no discolouration, swelling or any other sign of infection before you affix a new pouch. At all times, make sure no faeces comes into direct contact with the skin.

To dispose of the faeces, take the pouch to the toilet and cut the bottom of the pouch and empty the contents into the toilet and flush it. Take the plastic pouch and wrap it in newspaper or another plastic cover and throw it into the trash.

Approach the doctor if there is any discomfort, pain or change in the consistency or quantity of the stools.

13

Incontinence Management

What is incontinence?

Incontinence is just a large word for the lack of voluntary control over urination or defecation. Incontinence can be caused by medical conditions as well as age. Lack of bladder control is called urinary incontinence and the inability to control bowel movements is called faecal incontinence.

Faecal incontinence

Faecal incontinence is a condition where a person is unable to control their bowel movements, leading to stool leakage at unexpected times. It can be mild (such as a small amount leaking while passing gas, for example) or severe with total loss of bowel control.

Diarrhoea is a common cause for faecal incontinence and is easily managed through anti-diarrhoeal drugs. Another cause is constipation. Again, treatment of the underlying cause can help eliminate incontinence. For chronic incontinence, the most common cause is the weakening of the anal sphincter. This is the muscle that you control when you try and clench your anal muscles. If this is weak, it allows the leakage of some or all of the faecal matter collected inside. The weakening of the muscles could be due to various conditions including ageing, muscle or nerve damage, radiation, childbirth, surgery and rectal prolapse.

In addition, faecal incontinence can be caused by conditions such as dementia, Alzheimer's and other mental conditions that do not allow the patient to communicate their needs in a timely manner.

Urinary incontinence

Urinary incontinence is a condition in which a person is unable to control the flow of urine. It is also called involuntary urination. This condition is prevalent among the elderly, and more among women than men. This a problem that can affect active elders as well as those who are bedridden.

From a medical standpoint, there are four types of urinary incontinence. They are:

- *Stress incontinence:* This kind of incontinence is due to stress on the bladder. This can be triggered by coughing, sneezing, laughing, bending, lifting or other physical activity. It is common in women, especially among those who have given birth vaginally.

- *Urge incontinence:* This condition is sometimes referred to as an overactive bladder. A normal person feels the urge to urinate when their bladder gets half-full. At this stage, the brain tells the body that it would be nice if the bladder could be emptied, but there is no great hurry. As the bladder gets fuller, the brain keeps reminding the body at greater frequency until the bladder gets emptied. For people with urge incontinence, the brain starts asking the body to empty the bladder even when the bladder is nowhere near half-full. This is common in older men and women and is characterized by increased urinary urgency, an uncontrollable flow of urine and increased urinary frequency.

- *Overflow incontinence:* This condition is the opposite of urge incontinence. In this case, even when the bladder becomes full, the brain does not tell the body that it is time to urinate. Therefore, there is no urge to urinate. Consequently, the bladder overflows and a constant dribble ensues. Most often, this condition occurs due to a blockage in the bladder outlet or a narrowing of the urethra.

- *Functional incontinence:* This type of incontinence has very little to do with bladder-related issues. Instead, it is because the person is unable to reach a toilet in time for various reasons, such as a physical inability to move and/or communicate appropriately. This is prevalent among the elderly and people with diseases such as Alzheimer's or Parkinson's.

Based on the level of bladder control, or lack thereof, and the amount of urine that leaks, incontinence is classified as mild, moderate or severe. In the case of mild incontinence, only a few drops of urine may escape at a time. This could happen during the process of sitting down or standing up or while sneezing, coughing or making other sudden movements. Moderate incontinence is when there is leakage of more than a few drops of urine but much less than the full bladder's worth. Severe incontinence means that the person has very little control over their bladder, with most or all of the bladder contents leaking at one go.

As you can see, the reasons for incontinence are many. Thankfully, there are also many solutions, which we shall see shortly. The main message to take home at this juncture is that, no matter the reason, incontinence is eminently manageable and, in most cases, is not a life-altering condition for the sufferer.

Incontinence among active elders

Incontinence is a major problem if left untreated, especially for otherwise active people, and should not be ignored or trivialized. It is important to discuss this issue openly and provide support to the person suffering from this condition. Due to the embarrassing nature of the problem, most elders fail to bring it to the notice of family members or the doctor. Sometimes, they even refuse to acknowledge it to themselves. This can lead to a lot of problems for them and their family members.

As a way of managing this problem, many elders start by curtailing their activities instead of acknowledging and addressing the issue head-on. They become reluctant to go out which effectively results in a form of self-imposed house arrest. You will know this is happening when requests to go outside, even to a temple or a marriage, result in excuses such as 'I'm not feeling well' or 'I am too tired'. If you notice such a behavioural pattern emerging, do not treat it lightly. Have a talk with them one-on-one, or get a family member of the same sex who is close to them have a private talk with them. Failure to identify this problem early on will result in social isolation, which can lead to depression and other mental problems.

Managing incontinence

There are three main ways of managing incontinence. Depending on the underlying reasons for the condition, you can consider medical intervention and medication, exercise and physiotherapy, and/or use adult diapers and urinary pads.

The first thing to do is to consult a doctor, preferably a urologist or a urogynecologist. They will be able to identify the reason for the incontinence and guide you appropriately. Most often, incontinence can be managed with the use of adult diapers and pads. Sometimes, especially in the case of urge incontinence, pelvic floor exercises and bladder training can help. In some cases, medication that can help in regaining bladder control may be prescribed. In other cases, a medical procedure may be warranted. These medical procedures are predominantly laparoscopic and minimally invasive, so they do not require extended hospitalization and can be fairly inexpensive.

If your care recipient is bedridden, then you will definitely have to use a combination of diapers and underpads to maintain hygiene and reduce your work.

Diapers and their benefits

Adult diapers are pretty much the same as baby diapers, except that they are larger in size. A popular saying goes

like this: politicians and diapers have to be changed often
and for the same reasons! In this section, we will ignore the
politicians and learn about diapers. We will also outline
the ways by which you can determine what that 'often' is,
in terms of hours, in the case of a particular care recipient.

Adult diapers can be disposable or reusable. The
table below highlights the advantages and disadvantages
associated with both types.

	Advantages	**Disadvantages**
Disposable diapers	Hygienic	Mostly non-biodegradable; environmental pollutants
	Reduce chances of infection	Expensive in the long-run
	Available in the market	
Reusable diapers	Environment-friendly, non-polluting; biodegradable (usually)	Need to be washed and cleaned carefully; can otherwise lead to infections
	Inexpensive	Poor availability in the market

Since disposable diapers are more prevalent in India, we will look at those in more detail. Disposable adult diapers are not simple wads of cotton as one might imagine. They are fairly advanced products using new materials and polymers that make diapers comfortable to wear for extended periods.

Anatomy of a disposable diaper

Let us look at how a typical diaper is constructed. The topmost outer layer is usually a non-woven material that does not allow liquid to pass through. In most brands, these have a plastic-y feel, but some of the advanced brands have a cloth-like breathable material that allows air to pass through even though liquid cannot.

Under that is a layer of cellulose. This is a cotton-like fibre extracted from trees. Along with an inert polymer called the Super Absorbent Polymer (SAP), this layer forms the inner core. The SAP absorbs liquid and transforms into a gel, thereby ensuring that the core layer remains dry and there is no backflow when the diaper is squeezed. Once the SAP is used up, the diaper is said to be saturated as it will no longer be able to absorb any more liquid.

Finally, the innermost layer is a permeable material that is sometimes infused with anti-bacterial ointment that can prevent nappy rash. This inner layer allows the urine to flow through into the inner core so that the side that is in contact with the skin remains dry.

On the sides adjacent to the thighs are small elastic flaps that act as leak guards ensuring that urine does not spill out from the sides.

Finally, some diapers have lines on top that indicate whether the diaper is fully saturated and needs replacement. These wetness indicators are especially useful when the patient wearing the diaper is unable to communicate when the diaper starts feeling wet and needs to be replaced.

Choosing the right type

Disposable diapers come in two types—pants and nappies.

Pants-type diapers are like padded underwear with elastic at the top. These are largely meant for mobile adults and hence are easy to wear and remove. They are relatively thin and therefore very discreet, ensuring that it is not obvious to others when one is wearing a diaper. Another advantage of this diaper is that since it is easy to wear and remove, those that have access to a toilet have the option of using the toilet when available. The disadvantage is that because they are thin, the volume of liquid they can absorb is less when compared to a regular nappy-type diaper. It is important to note, however, that whether one urinates into the diaper or not, it is best to change it every eight hours or so.

Nappy-type diapers are thick and absorbent and usually meant for people who are essentially bedridden. They are a little difficult to put on by oneself, and usually one would require the help of another person to wear them. They have sticking tabs on both sides and have to be passed between the legs, wrapped around the waist and then stuck in place. The nappy-type diaper is ideally suited for people who need assistance, for those who are bedridden and those who require a diaper all night.

Selecting the right size

Once the type of diaper that is best-suited has been decided, the right size has to be chosen. Take the measurement of the waist. For many elders, waists would have disappeared, so use the navel as a guide and measure the circumference at that level. Each brand of diaper will have a size chart on their wrapper that shows what size should be chosen for a given waist size. Use this table to choose the right size. Some brands go by hip size, so it can be confusing at the beginning. If the initially chosen size doesn't work, try the next size. If even that doesn't work, switch brands.

Avoiding leaks

A leaking diaper is a lot of work and is best avoided.

There are two reasons for leaky diapers. One reason is choosing the wrong size. If the size is not right, urine may leak through the thigh area or the middle of the back. As the body shape for elders changes over time (for instance, the stomach area may get distended while the thighs may lose fat) from time to time, you may have to experiment with one or two brands and sizes before finding the best fit.

The second reason for leakage has to do with saturation of the diaper. As explained in the anatomy of the diaper section, a diaper can only absorb so much, beyond which it will start leaking. So, you will have to estimate the average outflow and then change the diaper before it gets completely saturated.

Incontinence and the bedridden

The best and most reliable way of managing incontinence among the bedridden is to use diapers and underpads. Not only do they keep the care recipient clean and dry, they also reduce the work of the caregiver significantly by reducing the number of times the sheets and clothes have to be changed.

Changing diapers

There are simple rules to follow regarding when and how often diapers should be changed.

When faecal matter is involved, it is best to change the diaper as soon as possible. Diapers do not handle faecal matter very well. While the liquid part of the faeces gets absorbed, the solid remains in touch with the skin. This can lead to a lot of problems if left unattended.

If you are looking after a bedridden loved one, here is what you can do to make life easier for yourself and them. First, try and set a routine if possible. Talk to your doctor and ensure that bowel movement is regular. If it is not regular by itself, controlled administration of laxatives under the supervision of your doctor can help regularize bowel movement. This can help in anticipating the time of the bowel movement and enables you to clean up at the earliest.

If that is not possible, then the only other option is the smell test. As soon as you smell faeces, change the diaper. Prompt action will ensure that infections are prevented.

As regards urine, a human bladder can hold a maximum of about 300–500 ml. A good diaper can hold about a litre. That should give you an idea of how often a diaper needs to be changed. Please remember that changes in medication can affect the output of urine. For example, diuretics can lead to excess urination. So, you may have to keep a regular watch on the medicines taken and appropriately modify the schedule for changing diapers.

For the average person who needs diapers all the time, expect to use at least three diapers a day. With a little discipline, you can set the schedule such that there are no midnight changes required. That way, the care recipient and the caregiver can have a good night's rest. Talk to your doctor, and they will help you figure out the liquid requirements of the care recipient and also help you taper the liquid intake gradually towards the evening in order to reduce the outflow during the night.

Importance of hygiene

It is very important to keep the abdominal and the pubic region clean to prevent rashes, allergies and infection. Failure to keep these regions clean and dry can lead to bedsores (pressure ulcers), nappy rash, fungal and bacterial infections and urinary tract infections.

Every time you change the diaper, use the opportunity to wipe down the area properly with wet wipes and let it dry before changing the diaper. Also, use this time to examine the patient for nappy rash and bedsores.

Use nappy rash creams liberally. The ones available for children are mild and non-allergenic and are also ideally suited for the elders' sensitive skin. Dust the area gently with talcum powder once in a while. However, unless there is a rash and the doctor has explicitly asked you to do so, do not apply powder in the vaginal and anal regions (perineal area). Do not put talcum powder directly on to the diapers as the powder will clog the pores in the diapers and prevent them from absorbing the urine.

Putting on and removal of diapers

Most diaper covers have detailed instructions on how to put on and remove diapers. For those using pants-type diapers, the wearing and removing process is a familiar one—just like using regular underwear—albeit with one difference. The final removal can be done by tearing the perforated sides and pulling out the diaper from between the legs, which makes the process much safer and easier. It is also a safe practice to wear and remove the diaper while seated rather than while standing. This will help in preventing falls.

As regards nappy-type diapers, the putting on and removal process can be a bit more cumbersome, at least initially, until one gets used to the technique. This is especially difficult—again, only initially—in the case of bedridden care recipients who are unable to help in any way. Having said that, the technique for changing the diaper is fairly simple once you get a hang of it.

If the care recipient is able to lift their hip at the required time, the process is trivial as you can expect. However, if the patient is completely immobile, then the process involves turning them on their side a couple of times. You can find videos on the Internet that demonstrate how one can change the diaper of a bedridden person efficiently.

Cleaning and disposal

Unfortunately, most disposable diapers are largely non-biodegradable. So, one can tell you to dispose of the diapers responsibly but, truth be told, there is no way one may actually be able to do so. However, here are a few tips:

If there is any faecal matter inside, please throw the faecal matter alone into the commode and flush it.

Roll the diaper as tightly as possible and store it somewhere where dogs, cats and various rodents cannot reach it. Then, when a few are collected, wrap them up tightly in some biodegradable cover and throw all of them into the dustbin. Eventually, one can hope they will get buried in some landfill, away from all of us.

Try and minimize the use of diapers as much as possible. That will be good for your purse and for the world!

Other incontinence products

Underpads

Disposable underpads are manufactured just the way diapers are, with the same layers, except that they are not shaped as diapers, but come in the form of sheets. These sheets can be spread on top of the topmost layer, usually the bedsheet, to absorb any excess urine that may leak out of the diaper.

You can change them when they get soiled.

Light incontinence pads

For people with mild incontinence, there are a lot of products available. These are smaller, less expensive and totally discreet. There are different models for men and different models for women. For the men, some of these models wrap around the penis and prevent drops of urine from soiling the underpants. For women, the pads are similar to sanitary napkins and used in the same way, except that they are designed to absorb urine.

14

A Safe and Secure Environment for Elders

Public spaces and office buildings in India are notorious for being senior- and disabled-unfriendly. Unfortunately, our homes are no better. The Indian home is probably about the most senior-unfriendly of homes anywhere in the world!

Though many of the houses are constructed with architects and engineers involved, there is scant attention paid to the special needs of the elderly who may live in those houses. Most doorways are narrow, hardly measuring 2.5 feet in width. The bathroom doorways are narrower still, sometimes measuring 2 feet or less. Why this is so is a big mystery. Pray tell, how much money does one save by shaving off a few inches from the width of the bathroom door?! The floors are uneven, and many times, the rooms are at different levels. Many homes with ground and first floors have neither bedrooms nor bathrooms on the ground floor, necessitating climbing stairs many times a day. The bathrooms are perennially wet, have slippery tiles and no grab bars to hold on to. Most rooms have projecting thresholds waiting to stub an unwary toe or, worse, trip a person.

Many multi-storeyed buildings have only stair access to upper floors as no provisions have been made for elevators. The steps on the stairs are steep, and in many places, the railing for the staircase is a cement wall that does not afford a firm hold. Taking a stretcher up and down these narrow stairways is a near impossibility.

To top it all, most Indian houses are cluttered with a hodgepodge of furniture collected over generations, making the house a veritable obstacle course for the less-than-agile senior citizen.

The list of what makes our homes unfriendly for its residents, especially the elderly and the disabled, is indeed a long one! You might feel that these are mere inconveniences, but if you have an unwell elder at home, each one of these 'minor' flaws can lead to serious problems if not addressed appropriately.

If your house is a typical Indian home, it is likely that you have at least some of these issues in your house too. Instead of trying to solve all of these problems, this chapter will endeavour to highlight what would be ideal, and then you can decide which problems to prioritize and which modifications you have the energy and budget to take on.

Bedroom comforts

With an unwell person at home, the bedroom becomes the room where most time is spent. So, a lot of care needs to go into making this a comfortable room for all those using it.

If you have the option, choose a room with a nice view of the outside. If your care recipient is bedridden, this will literally be their window to the world outside. Make sure there is ample sunlight coming in (at least during some part of the day) and there is sufficient cross-ventilation. A stuffy room can be gloomy and claustrophobic and can lead to depression. A room without sunlight can also lead to Vitamin D deficiency. If necessary, fit an air conditioner in the room so that you can control the temperature within, as summers in most parts of India can get really hot.

An attached bathroom would definitely make life easier for everyone. This is especially true when the care recipient is mobile and capable of walking to the bathroom and toilet by themselves. Get rid of all the unnecessary furniture, especially along the route from the bed to the bathroom, in order to reduce the chances of tripping while making their increasingly frequent and hurried trips to the toilet. Remove all stored items that are not relevant to the care recipient. The more stuff you have inside the room, the more crevices there are and the more dust will accumulate, making the work of keeping the room clean and dust-free that much more difficult.

There are also a lot of special furniture and gadgets that can make life easier for an elder at home. Some of them are listed below.

Cot

Choosing the right cot and bed can make life comfortable for the care recipient and the caregiver alike. In most circumstances, it is best to have a single bed for the care recipient. There is a wide range of cots and mattresses to choose from and it can be quite confusing at first. However, once you know what is required, for now and for the foreseeable future, one can make a well-considered decision.

The simplest cot is a standard 3 feet×6 feet single cot with a regular foam, spring or cotton mattress. For a mobile person requiring no special facilities, this should suffice.

However, for someone with limited mobility or for someone who may have breathing difficulties, you may want to consider what is called a Semi-Fowler cot. This is a cot that allows you to raise the head side of the bed, thereby enabling the user of the bed to recline at various angles.

If you need to have the care recipient's legs raised some of the time, then you can choose a Fowler cot. In this cot, the leg side can also be raised from the knee to the foot. For people with poor blood circulation or edema, it may be required that they keep their feet raised at least some of the time, and a Fowler cot can make it easy to position the care recipient appropriately without too much difficulty. Of course, most often, a Fowler cot is not really that important. One can always keep one or more pillows under the legs and feet to raise them.

There are also more sophisticated cots such as ICU cots that have more facilities. Some of these cots can be totally inclined in one direction or the other and can even be converted into a chair configuration.

All these cots come with optional caster wheels and need to have their own special mattresses that fold appropriately as the angles are changed. In addition, the cots come with a variety of side railings that ensure that the care recipient does not fall off the bed. You can get them in manual and electrical configurations. The electrical versions come with a remote that allow one to raise and lower them. These are very useful for bedridden patients who are capable of using the remote.

The cots used in hospitals are usually on the higher side because that is convenient for the doctors and nurses.

For home use, however, the cot should ideally be 18–20 inches in height (not including the mattress, airbed and sheets). This enables the care recipient to firmly place their feet on the ground when they are sitting on the edge of the bed, making it easier for the caregiver when helping them get off the bed. The headboard should be around a foot above the cot and the footboard at least 6 inches in height above the mattress level to ensure that the pillows don't slide off the bed.

If the care recipient is immobile or has limited mobility, ensure that there is enough space all around the cot to enable a person to move around freely. That way, you will have easy access to the care recipient from all directions. You will find this arrangement especially useful when two or more people are required for any manoeuvre.

The basic cot and mattress can cost from as little as Rs 10,000 to a few lakhs, depending on what is required. For most purposes, a basic Semi-Fowler should meet all your needs.

Bed-top and bedside tables

If the care recipient is confined to the bed for long periods of time, a few additional pieces of furniture can make life easier for everyone. One such product is a bed-top table. This is a small desk with 8–10 inch legs that can be placed on the bed and act as a table to rest a book on for reading or to keep the plate on while eating/feeding. You are sure to have seen one, if not in real life, at least in movies and advertisements where they depict someone being served breakfast in bed. There are a few models available in the market and most are foldable, so they can be stowed away when not in use.

Bedside tables are also an option. You can use them to keep medicines and some of the equipment you need regularly, such as nebulizers and phlegm suction apparatus. Some of these bedside tables can also be used as bed-top tables and can be used for serving meals.

Adjustable backrests

Adjustable backrests are also quite convenient to have around. If you don't have a Semi-Fowler or a Fowler bed, an adjustable backrest can be used on a regular cot to provide a way by which the care recipient can sit up with sufficient back support. Backrests provide a significantly more comfortable alternative to leaning against pillows bunched up against the headboard which can lead to backaches and neck pain.

Different models are available, with some to be placed under the mattress and others which are to be kept over the mattress. Most of them require a headboard or a wall to stay in place so that they do not slide off when leaned on. If a person is bedridden, an adjustable backrest is only a temporary solution. For proper support and comfort in the long term, it is recommended that you switch to using a Semi-Fowler or Fowler cot with an appropriate mattress.

Airbed

If the care recipient is lying down in the same position without moving for more than two to three hours at a stretch, then they are likely to get pressure ulcers, commonly known as bedsores. Pressure ulcers form when blood flow to some of the skin cells gets disrupted. When a person is lying or even sitting in the same position for long periods of time, some portions of their skin remain constantly pinched, thereby depriving some of the skin cells of much-needed oxygen. The cells then die, forming the nucleus of the ulcer. These ulcers can be very painful and may take a long time to heal.

An airbed, also called an alpha bed or an anti-decubitus mattress, can go a long way in preventing the formation of these pressure ulcers. An airbed is not just any inflated mattress. This device is a combination of a specially designed mattress and an electrical air pump. The mattress is made up of pockets or a series of tubes, and the pump constantly varies the amount of air in alternate pockets/tubes while it is operating, usually in a six- to ten-minute cycle. This ensures that the weight of the body is borne by different pockets/tubes at different points in time. Since no part of the body is constantly under pressure, blood circulation to all parts of the skin remains unimpeded, and thus ulcers are effectively stopped from developing.

The standard airbed is ideal for people weighing less than 100 kg. If the care recipient is heavier, make sure you ask for the heavy-duty model. To be effective, the pump has to be constantly on, which is fine as the pump has been designed to work 24×7. Obviously, you can switch it off if nobody is using the bed and switch it on about twenty minutes before the bed gets used again. Power consumption is extremely low, so you should not have to worry about the cost of running it.

Note that the airbed is not a replacement for the mattress but is meant to be placed on top of the existing mattress. Bedspreads, underpads and even rubber sheets can be spread on top of the airbed without affecting its efficacy.

If you are looking after a person who is confined to the bed for long periods, get an airbed installed at the earliest.

Remote bells

When one has an elderly person requiring support at home, the caregivers and family members need to be within hailing distance at all times. However, in a weakened state, the care recipient may not be able to raise their voice sufficiently to get the attention of those in the house. Under such circumstances, a remote bell is an ideal product to have.

A remote bell comes in two parts. One is the bell itself which can be fixed in any part of the house (from where you as caregiver will immediately be able to hear it at any time of the day or night) plugged into the mains. The other part is a small hand-held device with a single button that can be given to the care recipient or the primary caregiver sharing the room of the care recipient. This hand-held device is usually battery operated, and pressing the button will make the bell ring, thereby allowing the care recipient to draw the attention of people around whenever required.

Choose a bell that is not too jarring yet audible from anywhere in the house. Keep the bell portion as far away as possible from the care recipient (they are usually more sensitive to loud noises) while ensuring that they can also hear the bell ringing, so that they are assured that the bell is in working order. Keep the hand-held part within reach of the care recipient at all times.

Some family caregivers looking after a loved one tend to panic every time they hear the bell ringing. This need not be the case. If you are such a caregiver and the sound of the bell makes your heart race or leads to palpitations and sweating each time you hear it, please consciously learn to treat it as a non-emergency. Ask someone to ring the bell a few times so that you get over the urge to get into a frenzy every time you hear it ring. Learn to take your time, especially when you are woken up in the middle of the night (this will surely happen a few times) by the strident peals of the bell, because running around in panic when you are still groggy can be very risky for you.

Sometimes, the care recipient turns out to be trigger-happy and ends up pressing the bell very frequently for no reason. Under such circumstances, counsel the care recipient to use the bell judiciously. This may not always be possible, especially if the patient is suffering from dementia or some other form of neurological illness. Under such circumstances, you may not want to use the remote bell at all or, alternatively, you may want to keep it within reach only during certain times of the day when the care recipient is a little bit more capable of using their judgement.

Space to walk

One important aspect of the bedroom to consider at the time of equipping it for the elderly is the space required to move around without obstruction.

For mobile elders, the path to the bathroom from the bed is a frequently traversed one. In order to ensure that the care recipient does not trip, stub a toe, or bang their head on anything along the way, this path has to be made clear and easy to navigate. Remove all chairs, stools and other furniture that may come in the way. Also move or relocate all shelves, tables, bureaus and other furniture that may have sharp edges so that even if they were to fall, their head won't hit any sharp edges. If possible, and if the layout allows it, install grab bars in strategic places along the way so that the elder will always have something to hold on to when required.

If the person is largely confined to their bed in the room, arrange the cot in such a way that it is possible for a person to walk all the way around the cot. This will make it easy for one or more people to work together when moving the patient, changing sheets or administering medicines.

Lighting

The bedroom has to be well-ventilated, bright and airy during the day. During the night, depending on the condition of the care recipient, appropriate lighting arrangements will need to be made. If the care recipient is mobile, either there should be sufficient light for them to make their way from their bed to the bathroom without having to grope around in the dark, or there should be a night light and a switch within reach of their bed that would allow them to turn on the lights before leaving the bed. If the care recipient needs more support but not constant vigilance, then a dim light that is sufficiently bright is preferable. For elders requiring 24×7 monitoring, the room may have to be completely lit all the time. Care should be taken while positioning these lights so that they do not constantly shine directly into the eyes of either the caregiver or the care recipient when they are in their usual positions. Instead of using harsh incandescent bulbs, the room could be fitted with diffused lighting which is much more pleasant.

Attendant furniture

Quite often, people tend to ignore the needs of the attendant—be they a family member or hired help. With an unwell elder at home, it is only natural that all attention is directed at them. However, it is important to remember that only if the caregiver is healthy and attentive will the care recipient receive the necessary support and attention.

Depending on the needs of the care recipient, the furniture for the caregiver has to be selected appropriately. If the recipient requires constant attention and monitoring night and day, then a comfortable chair with an upright back ensures that the caregiver is comfortable but not sleeping. If the care recipient requires intermittent attention or is capable of asking for support when required, a comfortable recliner would be more suitable, allowing the caregiver to doze when possible, especially during the night shift. If the care recipient is fairly mobile and sleeps through the night, then an attendant cot (which can be folded and moved out of the way during the day) would be ideal, allowing the caregiver to also get a decent night's sleep.

Mosquito-proofing

If you live in a place that has mosquitoes, then one of the first things to do is to mosquito-proof the bedroom, if not the entire house. An already weakened immune system cannot hope to ward off the diseases borne by mosquitoes. Cover the windows with mosquito-proof mesh, have a second mesh door for the bedroom and keep a mosquito-killing racquet handy to take care of those that manage to get in anyway (there will be quite a few of these). Avoid using any chemical repellents for, in the long run, they are probably just as deadly to us as the diseases that the mosquitoes spread.

Alternative power source

Over time, depending on the needs of the patient, you may buy different equipment necessary to take care of your loved one. While many of the equipment require no power or run on batteries, some like oxygen concentrators and phlegm suction apparatuses require mains power. Since these service critical needs, if you are in a region that is prone to unscheduled power outages, you may want to consider an alternative power source such as a diesel-fuelled power generator for emergencies.

Other equipment

Taking care of someone at home is sometimes like running a mini hospital. Again, depending on the medical condition of the care recipient, the list of products that you will need may run from a handful to a list of twenty to thirty different products. Some of the more complicated equipment are described in greater detail in Chapter 11 titled 'Common Medical Equipment'.

Basic equipment

Some of the products listed in the beginning are available commonly in many households. Nevertheless, it may be a good idea to procure one more of these exclusively for the care recipient's use. A non-comprehensive list should include:

- Torch
- Emergency light

- Flask
- Measuring cups
- Dustbin
- Hand towels and a towel rod
- Stainless steel plates, glasses and spoons
- A source of clean water (a water purifier or an RO plant)
- Spittoons
- Hot water bottles
- Portable washbasins
- Paper dispenser

Consumables

- Wet wipes
- Dry wipes
- Sterile cotton
- Non-sterile gloves
- Face masks
- Hand sanitizer
- Diapers
- Underpads
- Syringes
- Catheter tubes
- Nappy rash cream
- Hand soap

Monitors and self-diagnostic equipment

- BP monitor
- Glucometer
- Pulse oximeter
- Thermometer
- Weighing scale

Advanced equipment

- Oxygen concentrator
- Nebulizer
- Phlegm suction apparatus
- ICU equipment

Making the bathroom senior-friendly

If you have ever perused home decor magazines such as *Architectural Digest* or *Better Homes and Gardens*, you would have seen photos of wonderfully designed, comfortable, opulent, dry and glistening bathrooms.

Unfortunately, these do not resemble Indian bathrooms in any way whatsoever. Most Indian bathrooms and toilets are small and ill-lit, have narrow doorways, have the slipperiest tiles on the floors and walls and are almost always wet. It is no surprise, then, that most of the accidents that happen at home happen in the bathroom, especially where senior citizens are involved.

However, with a few changes and some precautions, your bathroom can be made safe and usable. Most of the changes recommended here are cost-effective and do not require any major remodelling or masonry work.

Widen doorways

Let us look at some of the design issues first. The first thing you will notice is that the bathroom—referring to a bathroom, toilet or a combination of both—door is much narrower than the other doors in the house. It is usually 2 feet or less in width, making it impossible for most wheelchairs and commode chairs to pass through. Evaluate the feasibility of widening the bathroom doorway. This will make it easy for the elders and the caregivers to move in and out of the bathroom without unnecessary transfers, scraped elbows and fractured knuckles.

Put locks that can be opened from outside

The next thing you will notice is that the latch on the inside of the bathroom cannot be opened from the outside. With elderly people in the house, it is very likely that, at some point in time, the person inside may not be able to open the door by themselves and will need assistance from outside. Replace the latch on the inside with a door lock that can be opened from the outside in an emergency. Alternatively, you can replace it with a weak latch that will break easily on pushing. You may even remove the latch altogether and put a 'vacant/engaged' sign. This will allow people to quickly enter the bathroom if required as well as ensure that people know when it is occupied. This will cost very little and could save a life the next time an elderly family member has a dizzy spell or falls down in the bathroom.

Remember, the sooner you can reach a fallen or injured person, the greater their chance of survival and recovery.

Level floor

Another common problem with many Indian bathrooms is that the bathroom flooring is at multiple levels. In some extreme cases, the entire bathroom itself will be a good 6–9 inches above or below the rest of the house. In many more cases, where the bath and toilet are in the same room, the toilet will be at a level that is a few inches above the bathroom floor. Ideally, a bathroom floor has to be even and on the same level as the rest of the house. If that is not so, some masonry will help in levelling out the floor. This will prevent people from tripping as well as enable free movement in case the care recipient is wheelchair-bound. Most bathrooms have a small threshold that prevents water from coming out. This is fine to have as long as that threshold is less than 10 mm and has tapered edges.

Western water closet

A lot of old people cannot use the Indian-style toilet. If your toilet is an Indian one, there are commode chairs available that can convert them into Western commodes. However, these are temporary measures and are not convenient or hygienic. Convert your Indian toilet to a Western commode at the earliest. If you are making the modification, consider putting in one of the taller closet models and a health faucet or even an attached bidet.

With some of the corrective work out of the way, we can look at ways to improve the safety aspects of the bathroom further.

Slip-proofing the area

Indian bathrooms are perennially wet. The combination of a tiled floor (even if the tiles are anti-slip tiles) and water can make for a very dangerous situation. Add to that the talcum powder and oil often used in the bathroom and you have a veritable skating rink. A simple way to make the bathroom slip-proof is to put anti-slip mats on the floor. These are durable, low-maintenance PVC mats that can be laid out on the floor.

It is usually not required to cover the entire bathroom floor wall-to-wall as there are many spaces inside the bathroom that are not walked on, such as under the sink, behind the closet and under the taps where the buckets are placed. So, you can clearly mark out the areas where people are likely to walk and cover those areas with the anti-slip mat. Using brightly coloured mats can help the bathroom users know where to safely place their feet and which areas to avoid.

Grab bars, toilet raisers and safety rails

For many elders, even the standard Western commode is too low. If your elder one finds it painful to sit down or get up, you can fit a toilet raiser on the commode to increase its height. Additionally, you can also fix some grab bars on the walls nearby so that they have something to hold on to while getting up or sitting down.

If there are no walls nearby to screw on the grab bars, then you may want to get the type of toilet safety railing that can be easily fixed to the commode itself. This provides the same kind of support that the grab bars do. There are also safety railing models that can be just placed around the commode, requiring no bolting or grouting.

Shower chairs

Many people use a regular wooden or plastic chair for the purpose of sitting while bathing. This is not a safe practice as these chairs can break without warning, which can lead to serious injuries.

It is best if you can get a chair that has been specifically manufactured for this purpose. A wide range of such bath benches and shower chairs are available in the market. These sturdy, rust-proof chairs are usually height-adjustable and provide both comfort and safety.

Safety at home

Every day in newspapers across India there are articles about elders being targeted by thieves and crooks. Most often, these crimes happen inside the homes of the elders and result in the loss of cash and jewellery, minor to major injuries and sometimes even death.

Obviously, senior citizens living alone in their homes are easy targets for these anti-social elements. So, if your parents live alone or are alone most of the time when you are at work, then some precautions need to be taken.

The good news is, most of the thieves are only looking at the easiest targets, and even basic precautions can go a long way in ensuring safety of the elders. Here are some steps that you can take:

Have a grille door fixed

A majority of the people who come to your home are vendors and couriers who can be dealt with at the doorstep. If you have a grille door, then you can keep that locked permanently and just open the main door and make your transactions through the bars of the grille door.

If a thief comes home masquerading as an electricity board employee, a postman or a courier, all they can do is watch from the outside. Even if they ask for water to drink or something else that will necessitate you leaving them unsupervised, there is not much they can do when the entrance is blocked.

More often than not, they will go away to look for an easier target rather than think of how to gain access into your house. Remember, even the smallest efforts you take to keep yourself and your elder loved ones safe will go a long way in dissuading the potential thieves from trying to target your home.

Finally, if you have to let someone into the house (say, the gas man with a cylinder), then check their identity and credentials before you do so.

Don't keep valuables, jewellery at home

While you can keep most of the strangers out, it is not possible to keep everyone out. You still need to let the maids and housekeepers, various plumbers, electricians, doctors, nurses and nursing assistants into the house from time to time. While they are inside, they are bound to look around and notice things. If the people in the house are wearing a lot of jewellery, or if the deity in the pooja room is festooned with gold and diamonds, or they find money lying around within easy reach, they are bound to remember. And even if they are trustworthy themselves, they may mention it innocently in the presence of someone with malicious intent. If you don't keep such valuables around, people are less likely to look at you as a possible target.

Move your valuables into a bank locker. Wear simple cosmetic jewellery that no one can mistake for a genuine article. Keep as little money as possible in the house. Apply for and get a credit card from your bank. This can go a long way in reducing your need to keep cash around the house.

Proper lighting

Having proper lighting around the house can significantly improve safety in multiple ways. Proper lighting outside the house will allow you to see who has come in case of visitors after dark. Similarly, outside lights that are either on all night or that come on if there is movement can keep uninvited visitors away.

Inside the house, as already mentioned, proper lighting in the bedroom as well as in the rest of the rooms will help prevent people from tripping or bumping into furniture and walls.

Keeping friends and neighbours in the loop

As the world gets more connected, the neighbourhood seems to be getting more distant. We are constantly in touch with our friends and family, wherever in the world they may be, through WhatsApp, Skype and other software, but we don't even know those living next door to us.

If you have an elder person at home who may be alone some of the time, it is in your best interest to find out who your neighbours are. Build a nice rapport with them and ensure that you have a good relationship with them. That way, when you are not around, they will keep an eye on things happening around your house. In addition, they will be the ones providing company to the elders at home when no one else is around. This can also go a long way in staving off depression and dementia.

If the elder one is suffering from any neurological conditions such as Alzheimer's or dementia, then there is a possibility that they may wander off when you are not around. Having neighbours who are aware of the elder's condition will help in ensuring they don't go too far before someone in the neighbourhood spots them and brings them back home safely. There is no need to be shy or ashamed of accepting conditions like Alzheimer's and dementia. These illnesses are unfortunately fairly prevalent among elders, and keeping others apprised of these conditions is an absolute must.

Important phone numbers and speed dial

As people age, memory loss is common. Many times, even the most often-used numbers are forgotten. In order to ensure that elders at home have access to all the important numbers, print these numbers out in large font and stick them in one or two places around the house. In addition, most phones have a speed dial facility by which you can programme a few numbers to be called at the press of a single button. If your phone has a speed dial option, ensure that you put important numbers into it and teach the elders how to use them.

Important numbers include numbers of family members, friends and neighbours, the doctor, the nearest hospital, the regular pharmacy and those of other service providers.

Geofencing

With GPS devices available widely and most of the functionality for tracking becoming available in all smartphones, it is quite easy to track a loved one with the right device and software. Not only can you know their location at any given time with a high degree of accuracy, you can even set up a geofence (mark a territory) so that you are notified as soon as they step out of the territory. This way, if you suddenly find that your loved elder one has gone farther from their home than usual, you can take immediate action to guide them back home before they get lost or get into trouble.

Routines are important

Finally, if your loved ones live alone, it is important that some sort of routine be established. A routine that is recognizable by family and trusted neighbours, such as a good-morning call by phone at a certain time, a regular walk around the complex at the same hour, or even the sound of a pressure cooker at the same time every day, allows neighbours and family to unobtrusively find out that everything is normal at home. Also, any change in the routine will send an immediate signal for someone to quickly peep in and check if everything is as it should be, and if not, to take necessary action.

Additionally, cultivating 'good' habits is very important. As people grow older, they tend to forget things more often. Habits and routines help in ensuring that the important things get done consistently. Things like locking the door as soon as one enters the home, keeping the house keys and other objects in use (such as spectacles and money) in the same place, and writing down things in a notepad for ready reference will go a long way in providing a semblance of control over one's own life.

Kitchen comforts

Given that women in India spend a fair amount of time in the kitchen each day, one would think that it would be a fairly comfortable place for them to work in. However, this is not true. Thanks to the uncomplaining majority, the Indian kitchen is one of the most neglected rooms in the house when it comes to ergonomics.

Furniture

Indian cooking is a slow process requiring constant monitoring and ministrations, necessitating women to stand for long periods of time. Despite that, there is not a single comfortable high chair available in the market that would allow a person to sit and work comfortably at the kitchen counter. It may be a good idea to get one custom-made so that working in the kitchen becomes easier.

Safety knives and scissors

As people age, their grip becomes weaker. In addition, if the elders in the house suffer from tremors, this can make working with sharp implements quite dangerous. It is best then that people who may hurt themselves do not work with knives and other sharp instruments. However, if they are unable to avoid using these implements, it may be a good idea to buy them safety knives and scissors that are specially designed and manufactured for elders and children.

Safe floors

Some kitchens have a built-in wash area and/or leaky taps that make the floor wet. If your kitchen has a wet floor, it can lead to spills and falls that result in sprains, fractures or worse. You can either modify the kitchen or modify behaviour in order to ensure that the kitchen floor is always dry. If you can do neither, then at least put an anti-slip mat on the floor. Preventing falls is the best way of ensuring that elders remain active and independent till the end.

Preparing for emergencies

An emergency is defined as a serious, unexpected and often dangerous situation requiring immediate action. However, if you have an elderly person at home, emergencies should not be unexpected.

The type of emergency can vary depending on various factors, including the condition of the elderly person, the nature of accommodation and the area in which they live (rural or urban). Being prepared is half the battle. So, in this section, let us see what can be done to be prepared for emergencies.

Anticipate emergencies

Enumerate emergencies. Plan action to be taken. Prepare.

A first-aid event is an emergency. The patient could hurt themselves, or you as a primary caregiver could hurt yourself. Do you have an emergency kit ready?

A hospitalization event is an emergency. Read Chapter 6 titled 'Managing Hospitalization' for details on how to prepare yourself for such an eventuality.

There are other emergencies. The things that can go wrong with the city or town infrastructure are many. Power outages, stoppage of water supply, sewage getting backed up, *bandhs* and *hartals*, festive holidays with pilgrims overwhelming the infrastructure . . . the list is a long one. Do you have sufficient stock of all essentials to manage? Have you identified all the resources at your disposal in the case of an emergency?

Collate all important numbers

Make a list of all the important phone numbers, print a few copies in large font and keep them handy. You can stick the list in easily accessible places such as behind the door, on the insides of the cupboard door on the fridge door, and near the phone so that it is readily available to you. Make sure you have them in a language that is readable by the residents and caregivers. In case the caregiver is illiterate, put three primary contacts on speed dial on their phone and teach them how to use it. Ensure that the primary contacts have the list of important phone numbers ready.

Phone numbers should include primary contacts, neighbours, relatives and friends nearby, the doctor, the nearest hospital, the nearest ambulance service, the nearest pharmacies and so on.

Enlist support from friends, family and neighbours

In an emergency, you may require the help of others either to accompany you to the hospital, to look after the house, or for some other support. Rather than pouncing on them at the last moment, keep them briefed and prepared so that they are also primed for action. Assign each one of them a specific task you have in mind and let them know that it is their responsibility. Make sure they understand that they need to make alternative arrangements in case they are not available. That way, your support force is always ready for you when you need it.

Keep equipment handy

Basic emergency equipment such as a first-aid box, a working torch, candles, matchboxes should always be kept in readily accessible places. In the event of a power shutdown at night, you must be able to navigate your way to the torch without difficulty.

You must also have a set of house keys and, if you have a car, your car keys ready so that, in case you have to take your care recipient to a doctor, these keys are at hand.

Alternative power source

If you live anywhere in India, then you should be prepared for power outages. Apart from the basic emergency equipment listed above, you may also want to arrange for an alternative power source if required, especially if there is special equipment that needs to be available for the elder at home. Such equipment could include airbeds, suction apparatuses, nebulizers, oxygen concentrators, patient monitors and so on. Some of these may run on battery/inverter (low wattage items such as airbeds) while others will require a generator to function.

If a generator is required, ensure that it is wired and ready to use. Also test it regularly so you know it will start immediately when required. Needless to say, also ensure that it has enough fuel to power all needed equipment for at least twelve hours.

15

Mobility and Accessibility

Mobility (*noun*): The ability to move around (or be moved around) freely and comfortably.

Accessibility (*noun*): The quality of being easily reached, entered, or used by people who have a disability.

Mobility and accessibility go hand-in-hand. If you are mobile, most things are accessible, but as one's mobility diminishes, without forethought and planning accessibility diminishes too.

Before we go further, let us get this out of the way. Indian public and private places are terrible for the physically challenged. For those who are wheelchair-bound, India is surely hell. One could fill an entire book on all the places—both public ones such as banks, parks, roads and post offices as well as private ones such as our homes which we build using the services of architects and engineers—that are badly designed when it comes to accessibility.

To really understand how a disabled person might feel, hire a wheelchair for a day, sit on it and see how many of your normal activities you can perform. Then you will understand better.

In this chapter, we will try and understand some of the mobility-related issues elders face and appreciate their difficulties. We shall also see how we might be able to use the various equipment available to alleviate some of the problems associated with limited mobility and improve accessibility.

Acceptance and management

As people get older, their ability to move around freely and easily may be impacted adversely due to various reasons.

With age, muscles atrophy, bones become more brittle and one's sense of balance gets affected. Even a completely healthy elder can slowly lose the ability and the confidence to move around independently.

In addition, if there are other health issues such as, but not limited to, osteoporosis, arthritis, vertigo, or a recent surgery, then mobility can become a serious issue. Having said that, it need not be irreversible. Especially after an operation, with proper care and physiotherapy a person can regain most, and sometimes all, of their mobility.

There is also a kind of therapy called occupational therapy, though not many such therapists are available in India. An occupational therapist tries to understand the reason for the diminished mobility, figures out which muscles and capabilities are still strong and helps in retraining the body to learn again to perform many of the daily living activities with, if required, a different set of muscles. Though a lot of occupational therapy is focused on children, it can be useful in restoring independence to elders as well.

A lot of tools and standard equipment can also help in dramatically improving mobility. These include walking sticks, crutches, walkers and wheelchairs.

Choosing the right walking aid

The only elders who express an interest in buying a walking stick are those who need it to ward off stray dogs during their morning walks! Those that actually do need a walking stick because their legs are a little shaky, have vertigo, are losing their balance, or are not confident enough to walk on their own for some reason or another, find it very difficult to accept the fact that they need a walking stick to assist them.

For, indisputably, a walking stick is a symbol of old age, and no one wants to acknowledge the fact that they are getting old or that their body is no longer as young as it used to be.

This is a sensitive period for elders, a period where they will have to acknowledge their frailty, accept the situation, embrace a solution and, finally, resolve to continue to lead a life full of their favourite activities. This is not an easy process, and a lot of understanding and caring on the part of the caregiver is required to guide them along at this time and during times when they may have to graduate to a walker or even a wheelchair.

The single-leg walking stick

Though a lot of ornate wooden and metal walking sticks are available in the market, the ideal first walking stick is the inexpensive, height-adjustable, aluminium walking stick available at most senior citizens' stores and 'surgicals'. This walking stick may not be stylish, but it is functional and best-suited for the purpose.

Adjust the height of the walking stick for the comfort of the user. To find the right height, here are a couple of pointers. In their regular standing position with their hands hanging down by their sides, the walking stick's handle should be somewhere at the wrist level of the user. When they walk with the stick, check that their shoulder does not go up appreciably. If at the time they put the stick on the floor you see their shoulder going up, reduce the height of their walking stick by a notch or so.

There are lots of different walking sticks in the market, some of them functional as well as aesthetically pleasing. Wider bases, swivel mechanisms, shock-absorbers, reflectors and even inbuilt radios and GPS trackers are some of the features you will find on some of the advanced walking sticks. As long as they are height-adjustable and sturdy, you can buy any of them.

Some walking stick handles are made of soft (but firm) material while others come in hard PVC, plastic or metal. The softer handles are kinder on the sensitive skin of elders, so if there is a choice, go for the softer option.

There are also foldable ones available that are useful during travel as they can be packed into the bag or suitcase easily. These are ideal if the user is not putting a lot of weight on the walking stick. Otherwise, it is best to avoid them.

The tripod or quadripod

For those who need additional balance support, there are walking sticks with wider bases. The tripods have a three-pronged base while the quadripods have four. Either of these can be chosen as they both work the same way. The additional leg on the quadripod provides no greater advantage over the three-legged tripod. These walking sticks are free-standing, meaning that if you place them on the floor, they will remain upright without any additional support. They provide additional balance for the user.

Many first-time users tend to drag their wide-based walking stick behind them as though they are walking a dog on a leash. To use it correctly, one would have to take the walking stick and plant it in front of them so that it remains stable, and then hold it for support and move forward. This essentially makes the walk slower but safer. This means that the user needs to learn to consciously move slowly and methodically.

The crutch

The crutch is usually used by people who have sprained or broken one of their legs. There are two kinds. The ones you keep under your armpit are the regular crutches. The other kind is called an elbow crutch, which is like a walking stick with an additional extension that can be attached to the forearm. Most crutches are height-adjustable. Generally, these are not recommended for elders.

The walker

For people with significant balance issues, a walking stick may not provide sufficient support. What they might need is a walker. A walker has four legs widely spaced and allows the user to use both hands to hold it firmly and take steps.

Walkers are usually light-weight and height-adjustable. Most of them are also foldable, so they can be put away easily when not in use. There are several design variations:

- *The rigid walker:* This walker needs to be lifted and moved forward before each step is taken. The user will need to have the strength and coordination to lift the walker in order to use it properly. Consequently, one downside to this walker is that during the time the walker is being lifted and moved, the user will have to balance on their own.

- *The reciprocating-action walker:* This type of walker allows one to move the walker forward without having to lift it completely off the ground. Because it has a swivel mechanism, it allows one to move one side of the walker at a time, making the motion very similar to our regular walk. So, when you move the left hand forward, you can move the two left legs of the walker in front, and then you can move the two right legs together when you move the right hand forward. This kind of operation requires some coordination on the part of the user, but once they get used to it, it is very easy and convenient to use.

- *The wheeled walker:* The wheeled walker has wheels but only on the front legs. The back legs remain stumps. This walker can be pushed forward and requires the least amount of strength, effort and coordination on the part of the user. Many people worry that, because it has wheels, it may run away. However, since only the front legs have wheels, the walker remains in place until it is intentionally pushed forward.

  The only disadvantage to this walker is that on some floors, the back legs, which get dragged along the floor, may make a screeching noise that some sound-sensitive people may find annoying. Otherwise, it is completely safe and by far the easiest one to use.

- *The rollator:* This is the Mercedes of the walker world. It has wheels on all four legs, hand brakes, a seat to sit on when tired and even a small shopping basket under the seat. This is used mainly by people who are reasonably fit and well-coordinated but likely to get tired easily. You will find these rollators being used in large shopping malls by the elderly.

- *Hemi-walker:* There is also a special walker called the hemi-walker meant specially for stroke victims who have lost some or most of their control on one side. Unfortunately, this walker is not easily available in India.

Choosing the right wheelchair

For people who are unable to stand at all, there is no choice but to resort to the use of a wheelchair. For many elderly people, the process of accepting to use a wheelchair can be a traumatic one, so care has to be taken to gradually introduce the subject and involve them in the decision-making process. Springing a wheelchair on such a person may not be the best way forward.

Wheelchairs come in many shapes and sizes and with many features. Before you purchase a wheelchair, get a clear idea of how and when it is going to be used, how often and for what purposes. Also check whether the places where it is going to be used at are conducive for its use.

If the wheelchair is to be used within the house, then, at the minimum, the floors have to be level and even. The doorways, including those of the bathrooms, have to be wider than 32 inches, and the passages have to be able to accommodate the easy movement of the wheelchair.

Dimensions

Check the width, length, height and weight of the wheelchair when it is open and when it is folded. The inner dimensions will help you decide whether the size of the seat would be comfortable for the user, and the outer dimensions would help you confirm whether the wheelchair can be easily navigated around the house.

The folded dimensions and the weight of the wheelchair are needed to check whether it would fit in your car and whether the primary caregiver would be able to carry it when required. The weight of the wheelchair is of particular importance in cases where the primary caregiver is an elderly spouse. A lightweight wheelchair would definitely make life easier for them.

Most wheelchairs available in India are certified for people weighing less than 100 kgs. The bariatric ones can handle up to about 125 kgs. If your care recipient is heavier, you may have to either get a wheelchair commissioned locally or have a special one imported.

Manual vs motorized

A manual wheelchair is one that has to be pushed to be moved. If the person using the wheelchair has sufficient upper body strength, you can get a wheelchair with large rear wheels. These allow the user to propel themselves around. In case the user does not have sufficient strength in both arms or is incapable of self-propelling for other reasons, it may be best to get an attendant wheelchair. These have smaller rear wheels and therefore are of narrower width and thus are easier to manoeuvre for the attendant.

A motorized wheelchair is a battery-operated wheelchair with a joystick that lets the user drive around. These are usually expensive, heavy and difficult to use inside most Indian homes. So, unless you have an unusually large house that is well-designed with wide passages and doorways and/or live in a location that is wheelchair-friendly, such as a safe, gated community with wide pavements that are even and obstacle-free, getting a powered wheelchair may not be such a good idea. If you do decide to buy one, ask the company to bring one for a demonstration and try it out for real.

There are basically two types of motorized wheelchairs available in India. The first type is a regular manual wheelchair, mostly imported, that is locally retrofitted with motors and batteries. All motorized wheelchairs are expensive, but this kind is comparatively less so. Though it will work as expected, its performance will necessarily be subpar. The second kind is a powered wheelchair that has been built from the ground up. While some of these are manufactured in India, most are imported, mainly from China. These are usually of better quality and, naturally, more expensive. You can actually buy a small car for the price of some of the high-end, powered wheelchairs.

Selection process

In addition to manoeuvrability, you may have other requirements for the wheelchair. For example, you may want it to be comfortable to sit in for long periods of time, or you may want it to double as a bedside commode or even as a shower chair. Thankfully, a lot of people have been giving thought to all aspects of wheelchair-based existence and have designed and manufactured literally thousands of wheelchairs with diverse functionalities, including some that will help the user move from a sitting position to standing upright and back. The flipside is that you now have a problem of plenty. In order to make it easy for you to make a decision, get answers to some or all of the following questions:

- Is the wheelchair for indoor use or outdoor use?
- Do you want a manual one or a motorized one?
- Should it be a self-propelling version or an attendant wheelchair?
- Does it have brakes?
- Is it rust-proof? Is it waterproof? Does it need to be?
- What are its dimensions and will it enter your bathroom doorway easily?
- What is its weight capacity?
- How much does it weigh? Can you lift it easily?

- When folded, does it go into the boot of your car?
- Are the armrests removable? Are the footrests removable?
- Can the upholstery be changed?
- Will it be comfortable to sit in for long periods of time?
- Does it have a commode attached? Can it be used as a shower chair?
- Is it easy to clean?
- Does it have the facility to recline?

There may be other such questions that are unique to your needs. Write them down before you go to select a wheelchair for a loved one. In many ways, it is like buying a car. It is important to buy one that meets most of your current needs as well as those that might arise in the foreseeable future.

Here is a short note on wheelchairs that come with a commode attachment. These are very tempting to buy when you have a bedridden patient at home as they can dramatically reduce the amount of discomfort the patient will have to bear (and the amount of heavy lifting the caregivers have to put in).

The typical morning hygiene routine goes as follows:

- Get the patient to sit up in bed.
- Transfer them to a wheelchair.

- Move them to the bathroom for toileting and bathing.
- Move them from the wheelchair to a commode chair.
- Move them from the commode chair to a bathing chair.
- Move them from the bathing chair to the wheelchair.
- Transfer them back from the wheelchair to the bed.

As you can see, there are a total of five transfers to be made. This can be truly back-breaking, as anyone who has been around bedridden people can attest, for the human body is extremely unwieldy. A wheelchair that can double (or triple, actually) as a commode chair and shower chair could easily reduce the number of transfers to just two—from bed to wheelchair and back.

However, a typical wheelchair (one which is primarily a wheelchair) with a commode attached is not the ideal choice, especially when it comes to hygiene issues. They usually have lots of folds and crevices, maybe wheels with spokes, and this means that dirt and faecal matter have a lot of places where they can get irretrievably lodged, and that is definitely not desirable. In addition, these wheelchairs with commodes come with hard seats which make sitting on them for extended periods uncomfortable, to say the least.

Nevertheless, having a wheelchair that can work as a commode and shower chair is very much desirable.

So, go for one that is a shower chair and commode chair with wheels. These are usually designed with hygiene in mind, and the wheels are sufficient to move the patient around from bed to bath and back. For transportation purposes, get a separate wheelchair that is more suited for that purpose.

Usage

There are a few simple instructions to keep in mind while using a wheelchair so that the person sitting in it remains safe and comfortable:

- Whenever you are moving a person in and out of the wheelchair, ensure that the brakes are on. You do not want the wheelchair to move away when the person is about to sit on it or get up from it.
- When the person is seated, ensure that their legs are firmly placed on the footrests. Also ensure that before the person gets up, the footrests are moved out of the way. Care should be taken to ensure that the person does not step on the footrests when getting up as that would topple the entire wheelchair.
- Ensure that the person's elbows are firmly inside the armrests when you are moving them around. Make sure that they are not on the armrests or dangling

outside the armrests. This will prevent them from inadvertently bumping their elbows against walls and door frames.

- Always ensure that the seatbelt is firmly fastened.
- When you are moving them around on a surface that is not even or smooth, take your time and move slowly. The front wheels of most wheelchairs are small and can easily get stuck in depressions and protruding ledges. When that happens, the wheelchair can easily topple forward, upending the occupant. This can lead to grievous injuries, especially to the face, palms and knees.
- While moving up an incline, push the wheelchair as you normally would with the wheelchair in front and you at the back. However, while coming down an incline, do it in the reverse. Imagine a video of you going up the incline but being played in reverse. You will be behind the wheelchair but you will be walking backwards slowly, with the wheelchair and its occupant facing away from the direction of movement.

Accessibility in the house

In addition to using physiotherapy, occupational therapy and equipment to improve mobility, you can also rearrange and redesign your house to make the care recipient more independent. We have looked at some of these aspects in Chapter 14 titled 'A Safe and Secure Environment for Elders'.

Some of the simple activities that we take for granted (such as turning on and off lights and fans, brushing our teeth, combing our hair, shaving) can become difficult for a person with limited mobility. Instead of making them feel dependent, we can use simple technology to make them more self-sufficient.

To begin with, you can move all the switches to be within reach. If that is going to be difficult, you can change the switches to those that support remote operations. A lot of smart switches are available in the market, and one remote control unit can be used to operate a whole range of switches very easily.

You can also change the design of the taps and door knobs to be easy to grip instead of the models that are round and smooth and difficult to hold. This will enable a person with arthritis or weak hands to operate these knobs without external help.

If you cannot change these (for example, if you live in a rented place and the owner does not allow you to), there are rubber grips available that provide additional traction to all these knobs.

Small indoor and outdoor elevators are available, and these can be installed without too much reconstruction. These will enable the mobility-impaired person to gain access to other floors in the house. If this is not possible, there are chair lifts available. These run on railings on your existing stairs, so a person can sit on the chair lift on the ground floor and use the powered system to move up along the rails to the next floor.

Where a few steps may prevent wheelchair access to areas, a small ramp (either permanent or movable) can be constructed to provide access. There are clear specifications with respect to the dimensions of these ramps available on the Internet which will help you ensure that the incline is not too steep.

Accessibility outside the house

Unlike in developed countries, public places in India are not designed after taking into consideration the needs of the disabled.

So, when you take your mobility-challenged elder out of the house—for a doctor's visit, to the hospital, to a wedding, a mall, a theatre, or a holiday—you need to check on a few things beforehand in order to ensure that you are able to look after their comforts properly when outside.

Elevator access

Check that the place you are going to has elevator access if it is not on the ground floor. Check if the elevator is large enough to accommodate a wheelchair and an attendant. You might think that it is a silly question, but there is a retirement community building in Chennai where the lift is so small that it cannot take in a standard wheelchair. So, don't take anything for granted.

Ask if there is a backup power generator for the elevator in case there is a power breakdown.

Ensure that you don't have to climb up or down any steps to reach the elevator. This is strangely the case in many buildings. Typically, the elevator will be in the lobby and the lobby will be a few steps above ground-level. There are even hospitals where this is true. One way to avoid the steps is to go to the basement and get into the elevator from there. Most often, especially where there is a basement car park, the elevator begins there, and since it is a car park, there will be a ramp that leads down to the basement.

Toilets

Bladder issues are practically unavoidable for the aged. Elderly people need to have ready toilet access, usually on an urgent basis. If you are taking your elderly parent(s) to, say, a wedding, you will need to seat them within easy reach of the toilet. If any of them is wheelchair-bound, you will also need to check if there is a disabled toilet in the marriage hall.

Alternatively, get the elder to wear a diaper. Just the confidence that the diaper brings will give them and you more time to reach a toilet when needed.

Wheelchair availability

Check if the place you are visiting has wheelchairs available for use. Take your own, otherwise. Most major cities have companies that hire out wheelchairs, so you don't necessarily have to buy one if it is only for occasional use.

Travelling

In the case of local or intercity travel, prepare to travel by car. That way, you can plan timely breaks and make the journey as comfortably as possible.

Travelling by train can be difficult. Keep in mind that to get into and out of Indian trains, one is required to navigate a ladder. This can be very difficult for older people. Also, if the lower berth is not available, it can be downright dangerous for elders to try and climb onto the middle or upper berths.

As for bus travel, the less said, the better. Sitting for long periods in cramped seats can create a lot of health issues anywhere in the world. On top of that, if the journey is bumpy, thanks to bad roads, there is no way it can be made comfortable. Also remember that overnight buses may not stop for bio-breaks at regular intervals. And even when they do, the toilet facilities at these stops may not be clean enough to use.

Air travel, however, is a good option. Most airports are easy to navigate and quite senior-friendly. Also, most airlines provide wheelchairs on request, which is a blessing.

Unfortunately, many Indians misuse the wheelchair facilities at airports. Next time you are flying somewhere, do notice the number of elderly but fit men and women who use wheelchairs they don't need. It's because their children believe that they are incapable of moving from one terminal to another. They also know that, as an added benefit, transfers become easier, thanks to knowledgeable attendants who know their way around the airport. It is both funny and sad to watch a perfectly capable elder jump off the wheelchair at the gate and traipse into the aeroplane!

Please request for a wheelchair for your loved one only when necessary. Understand that there are only so many wheelchairs available and someone with a genuine need may be waiting for it.

16

Retirement Communities

Breaking the taboo

Till a few years ago, for the average Indian, the term 'Old Age Home' only brought up disturbing images of destitute homes run by charities and populated with homeless people. In our country, the phrase is still closely associated with a lot of negative connotations such as desertion, depression, destitution, dearth, disease and death.

It is true that until recently, old age homes were as you imagined them to be—just another name for destitute homes. After all, only the poor needed them. The rich had their money, their palatial homes, their connections with doctors and an army of servants to look after them. As for the majority—the middle class—they were too busy trying to get upwardly mobile to worry about ageing issues. Besides, the joint family structure prevalent till a few decades ago cushioned them from many of the problems today's nuclear families are facing.

Now, the world is changing. People in the middle class are now a little richer, wealth-wise. Simultaneously, they have also become poorer in terms of quality of family life due to the loss of the supportive joint family system. Healthcare has improved, enabling people to live longer, more active lives. At the same time, it is also prolonging the life of the infirm without substantially improving their quality of life. To add to the complications, the search for a challenging career and a better life is taking grown-up children to faraway places, forcing more and more older people to live by themselves.

To counter this upheaval, the burgeoning middle class' attitude towards old age homes—now called retirement communities—should also change and keep up with the times. Retirement communities are becoming a necessity now, and if you wish your elders to be comfortable in their later years, you must embrace this concept wholeheartedly.

A retirement community can enable your elder loved one to lead a safe, secure and comfortable life. The retirement communities that are coming up today to meet the demands of the middle class are designed to provide a lot of facilities that you would be hard-pressed to find in standalone homes or regular apartments. These include enhanced security, healthcare, companionship and help around the house, to name a few.

Our job should be to dispel our prejudices and embrace these new-world solutions to our new-age problems. Many elders have already moved into such homes and are paving the way for wider acceptance within our population.

Types of retirement communities

The Indian retirement community industry is still in its nascent stages. The facilities provided are not yet comprehensive and nowhere near the standards set by those in the Western world. But we are getting there fast.

This section introduces you to various types of retirement communities, some of which are yet to emerge in India. However, knowing what is available elsewhere will provide you with the ammunition needed to demand such facilities so that we can all get these facilities here in India, sooner rather than later.

Worldwide, there are four broad categories of retirement communities. These categories are based on the level of independence the residents have as well as the nature of services provided to them. The categories are: independent living communities, serviced living communities, assisted living communities and continuing care facilities.

Independent living communities

Independent living communities are for elders who are healthy, independent and mobile. These communities are similar to regular gated communities with basic facilities such as security, power backup and building maintenance support.

The difference is that, in addition, they are built to certain specifications that make them suitable for elder living. For example, all places within the community are made accessible by ramp or elevator so that no stairs have to be taken. All the doors in the dwelling (including bathroom doors) are built to be at least 32 inches wide, allowing for easy wheelchair access. Bathroom doors are designed to be openable from the outside in the case of an emergency. Wet areas, toilets and bathrooms are provisioned with anti-slip tiles with rough surfaces and/ or anti-slip mats as well as grab bars that help in safely navigating around the bathroom and easing sitting down and getting up from commodes and bath chairs. Finally, these places are built close to medical facilities with ambulance services.

Serviced living communities

Serviced living communities are also built for healthy, independent and mobile elders. However, in addition to providing all the facilities that the independent living ones provide, these provide some or all of the following services:

- **Food:** Many communities have a common kitchen and dining area where standard fare is prepared and served. Those residents who don't wish to cook anymore can use these facilities as and when they wish. As we all know, the typical Indian woman in a traditional home never retires because she has to cook for the household throughout her life. This service provides an opportunity for the Indian woman to eliminate kitchen work, if not every day, then at least on some days.

- **Laundry and housekeeping services:** With age, even simple tasks involving manual labour become more and more difficult. Having hired help can alleviate some of these problems, though managing them can still be a challenge, what with 'no shows', festival bonuses and sundry demands. By taking on the task of providing housekeeping services, the management of these communities take this burden completely off the shoulders of the residents.

- **Medical support:** Serviced living communities provide some or all of the following medical services, including a doctor-on-call available within the community, access and some kind of tie-up with one or more nearby hospitals providing special, speedy and preferred processing for the residents, ambulance facility, local nursing and nursing assistant support, regular medical check-ups, and management of medical records and medical insurance.

- **Programmes and activities:** While there are huge benefits to living in a single-demographic retirement community, it can get tiresome too with only old people talking about health issues for company. To compensate, many communities have a dedicated activities manager who ensures that there is always something interesting happening within the community so that the varied interests of residents are catered to. From joint prayer sessions to evening concerts, from yoga sessions to potluck dinners, a good activity manager can keep the entire community buzzing and happy.

- **Concierge services:** Many elders travel widely these days. This is a new trend among the active elders in India, and an in-house concierge service can help make the necessary arrangements. Over and above being a travel agent, these service providers are also sensitive to the needs of the travelling elders, such as their accessibility requirements, diet restrictions and preferred modes of travel. This knowledge and sensitivity makes them capable of chalking out senior-friendly travel plans that can make travelling truly pleasurable.

Assisted living communities

Assisted living communities are for elders who are less than independent. They are designed for elders who need assistance to complete the daily living activities, to those who may need 24×7 care but short of requiring hospitalization.

In addition to all the services provided by serviced living communities, assisted living communities provide support for daily living activities and nursing care, medication management, physiotherapy, occupational therapy, memory care and regular medical supervision.

Unfortunately, there are not very many facilities that provide this level of service in India yet. Most of the existing retirement communities fall in the first two categories. So, if you have a wheelchair-bound or bedridden patient who is otherwise stable, or an Alzheimer's patient or someone with some other form of dementia, you have very few options other than home care.

Medical insurance also does not cover this kind of service in India, so the costs involved in any kind of retirement community living will have to come from the savings of the elders or their children.

Continuing care communities

Continuing care communities don't yet exist in India. These are communities which provide all the levels of service outlined above, under one roof. One can move in when fully independent, say, into an independent villa and then transition within the same community to other types of accommodation based on the changes in one's condition. So, as one ages, one may move from an independent villa to an apartment, and then to a single room with nursing care, all under the same agreement.

This is a truly wonderful arrangement when it works. Unfortunately, this kind of facility is unlikely to be available in India for the foreseeable future.

What to look out for

Once you have decided that moving to a retirement community is an option, it is time for a thorough due-diligence exercise.

The first thing to know is that, as of now, a retirement community is not an option if the elder loved one is bedridden. For that, there is no option but home healthcare. One or two alternative options are coming up, but without insurance cover, these may be quite unviable.

If the elder ones are mobile, independent and willing, then it may be possible to find a nice retirement community that meets their requirements. If not for ever after, at least for as long as they are mobile, independent and willing.

Understand the promoter

Begin the process of scrutiny by understanding the background of the promoter of the retirement community. If it is a realty company, they are probably just using the phrase 'retirement community' to attract the senior citizen segment. If they are planning to build, hand over and move on, then the project is just another regular housing project. Steer clear.

If the promoter has an operations background (having run a retirement community or a hospital or even a hotel before) and provides operational plans for the foreseeable future, then you are on a good wicket.

Location

The location is very important. Check how far the nearest health clinic is. Find out which are the most accessible multispeciality hospitals and how long it would take to reach them. Once the elders are there, the family might want to visit, so check how easy it is to reach the place. Is it within city limits? If not, which is the nearest airport, railway station or bus stand? How long would it take for the elder residents to reach the city of their choice?

Heterogeneity

Some elders prefer to spend time with others of the same age group. Some others would want to live in a mixed environment where they can see and interact with younger people. Check if the retirement community is a dedicated elder community or an integrated facility. In many cities now, the builder plans for, say, ten towers of apartments and hands over one or two of them to a retirement community operator. This operator then redesigns the apartments to be senior-friendly (which can be done well if they get involved before the construction begins) and provides services to help elders lead a comfortable life. This is quite a nice approach and provides all the facilities one expects from a retirement community while also ensuring that the residents are part of a real-life multi-demographic integrated society.

Ownership

Understand the ownership options. While most retirement communities require you to buy the dwelling units, some do have other options, such as long-term and short-term leases as well as rental options. There are pluses and minuses to each of these options.

While outright ownership has its advantages, it also means that you are making a long-term commitment. Moving out if the facility proves unsuitable can be difficult. Long-term and short-term lease options are ideal though hard to come by. Basically, these facilities ask you to pay a moderate amount as an interest-free, returnable deposit. Once you have made that deposit, the dwelling is as good as yours for as long as you want it. And when you vacate, they return the deposit to you. Of course, you will still have to pay for all the services you use during your stay. This model is ideal because it gives you the right to stay as if you were the owner as well as provides you with the option to move out easily if and when you choose to. The only concern with this model is the reliability of the service provider and how sure you are that they would be in a position to return the deposit when you leave. If the provider has a reliable track record, is backed by a well-known brand or a bank, or some other reliable institution is involved in the agreement as a guarantor, then you should be safe.

Outright rental options provided by the community administration are rare. However, in every retirement community, there are dwellings purchased by people who, for some reason or the other, are unable to live there. If , you can identify them, then you could approach them to rent the apartment/villa to you. Many of the community administrators themselves support this model, so you could even approach them directly and check if they know any owners who have apartments for rent. The downside is that if the owner decides to move in, you will have to vacate.

Size and configuration

Understand the types of residential units available. As already mentioned, most retirement communities in India provide only a buy-and-live model. So, the decision on the type of residential unit is very important as you cannot move as easily as if you were only renting the place. Many of the up-and-coming retirement communities provide independent houses (ostentatiously called 'villas') as well as apartments of various dimensions to suit the budget and privacy needs of its residents. Visit the project, understand the layout and choose wisely. While an independent villa sounds nice, it has its own set of issues. It may be too big to manage, or it may become progressively difficult to get to the dining area, for example, if it is a little far away. Remember, the residents may have to make this trip thrice a day, whatever the weather, so even a short walk may be too far away on some days. Additionally, if the planning isn't very good, some of these villas may be two-storeys high, necessitating the climbing of stairs.

Apartments, though they may not be as exclusive and luxurious as villas, offer other benefits. The common facilities are more easily accessible, and a smaller area, if it is only for one person or a couple, is much easier to manage and maintain. They are also easier on the purse.

Some retirement communities also provide individual rooms with attached bathrooms either for single occupancy or on twin-sharing basis. For elders needing support in their daily living activities, this is a good option as help is always at hand and the distances needed to navigate are limited.

Services

The services provided by the retirement community should be the most important criteria in helping you decide which retirement community to choose. Some so-called retirement communities will tell you that they will operate the facilities for X years, after which the residents' association is expected to take over. Give these a pass. They are realty players masquerading as retirement community operators.

A reliable retirement community operator should provide a menu of services and levels of services to choose from along with clearly stated costs associated with each of them. Depending on whether they are an independent living, serviced living, or assisted living facility, the number of menu items could range from a few items to a comprehensive list of over fifty services. Understanding this list should give you an idea of what to expect and what the monthly budget will come to, per person.

Here is a checklist of services for your ready reckoning:

- *Accessibility and safety*

  - Are all areas accessible? Are ramps and elevators available to make access easy?
  - Is the flooring level inside the dwelling unit?
  - Are the floors slip-proof? Are the bathrooms and wet areas slip-proof?
  - Are all the doors, including bathroom doors, wide enough for wheelchair access?
  - Are grab bars and shower seats provided in the bathrooms and toilets?
  - Are the locks on the main door, bedroom doors, as well as the bathroom and toilet doors operable from outside in case of emergencies?
  - Are Western toilets fitted? Are they 19–20 inches in height?
  - Are there easily accessible emergency-calling facilities within the dwelling?
  - Is there adequate lighting within and outside the dwelling unit?

- Are there telephone facilities with extensions in bedrooms and bathrooms?
- Is there 24×7 security? Are video doorbells available?
- Is there immediate access to emergency aid and ambulance services?
- Is there a nearby hospital with house-call support?
- Is there guaranteed power backup?

- *Infrastructure and maintenance*

Most regular gated communities provide general upkeep services. So, while these should go without saying, it is always better to ask and confirm the availability of the following:

- Captive plumbing, electrical and general maintenance services
- Gardening and upkeep
- Security services
- Internal transportation facilities

- *Resorts and serviced apartments*

Most retirement communities come up outside cities and towns as the land cost is cheaper in these areas. This gives these promoters additional budgetary freedom to add some useful features. Check out if they have:

- Guest accommodation so that visitors can come and stay for a few days without burdening the ones they are visiting.
- Serviced apartment management services for visitors staying longer.
- Resort-style services which will incentivize families and grandchildren to visit.

- *General household services*

Most elders would be happy to be freed from mundane tasks such as those around the house. After all, that time could be spent better pursuing hobbies or even just snoozing. Check whether the following services are provided:

- Laundry services
- Linen services for changing the sheets and curtains on a regular basis
- Housekeeping

- *Personal services*

Just like everybody else, elders too have the need to look good and stay healthy in order to be happy. Check to see if at least some of the basic facilities listed below are available within the community itself:

- Grooming services
- Regular medical check-ups
- Pets support services (pets can provide love and companionship and help in keeping depression at bay.)

Concierge services

Just because one is in a retirement community does not mean that life as one knew it is over. A lot of older people with money and time on their hands have started travelling regularly, especially to senior-friendly destinations abroad. An in-house concierge service would go a long way in finding destinations and making the arrangements. Check to see if they offer the following services:

- Travel desk to arrange for local transport to go into town, catch a movie or concert, or go shopping
- An agent for ticket booking and hotel reservation
- Appointment booking with doctors, spas and salons
- Bill payment service
- Travel desk for longer vacations

Catering services

It is said that an Indian woman can never retire because the kitchen is never closed. For women, the single compelling reason to move into a retirement community is escaping the drudgery of cooking all meals every day. Even if they love cooking, they will appreciate the option to not cook on days when they don't feel like it. Most serviced and assisted retirement communities provide a common canteen that serves all meals. Of course, residents can continue to cook their own meals if they wish to. Check for the following facilities:

- Canteen services and common dining area
- Kitchen within the dwelling unit
- Restaurant-type dining with an a la carte menu
- 24×7 coffee shop
- Room service
- Special menu services (Jain food, vegan, diabetic-friendly)
- Non-vegetarian food
- Bar

Entertainment

Many retirement communities also have full-time event managers to keep elders busy and joyfully occupied. Some facilities and services to look out for while choosing retirement community for your loved one are:

- Activity management
- Concert and movie ticketing

- Library and magazine service
- Programmes and activities
- Senior gym
- Space for gardening

Assisted living services

If the elders are less than fully independent, you will need to look for additional services over and above what has been listed already. Check for:

- Ambulation and companionship services
- Nursing assistance (changing diapers, Daily Living Activity [DLA] support)
- Nurse on call
- Periodic key health parameter-monitoring, tailored for each individual based on their state of health
- Medication assistance
- Medical records management
- In-house doctor
- Emergency services
- Ambulance services
- Tie-ups with nearby hospitals for preferred treatment
- Periodic medical screening camps
- Diabetes care
- Physiotherapy, occupational therapy
- Hydrotherapy

17

Importance of Sex and Companionship

According to a recent study conducted among Indian seniors regarding their sexual lives . . . Who are we kidding?! No such study has likely ever been conducted. Who would have the temerity to ask elders questions about their sexual proclivities in this staid country? After all, most of us believe elders don't care about sex. Come to think of it, some of us don't even believe our parents have ever had sex at all!

Given this blinkered view of life, it is no wonder that scant attention is paid to the physical and emotional needs of elders.

While we may not have many studies conducted in India, there are quite a few that have been done in Western countries. All of them show that most elders are fairly active sexually, well into their 70s and even 80s and beyond. In fact, a study conducted in old age homes in the US—yes, the kind that brings up images of really old people doddering around with the help of walkers and staring blankly at television screens—showed that sexually transmitted diseases were rampant in these establishments. This proved that the residents were having sex regularly and with multiple partners. The STDs, of course, spread because none of them used condoms, for after all, who was going to get pregnant there?

Shocking? Not really; at least it shouldn't be. Just because we have buried our heads in sand does not mean it is night-time, does it? So, it is time to face the truth. There is every possibility that Indian elders, who are no different from elders anywhere else in the world, may have the same urges and needs as their counterparts elsewhere in the world.

Anyway, to put your mind at ease, just remember that sex and intimacy do not have to necessarily mean the whole act, all the way, all the time. Companionship, holding hands, sleeping together (literally) and cuddling are all intimate acts that can improve the health and well-being of people across all ages, including those entering their sunset years.

Making a beginning

When those Indians who are now in their 40s and 50s enter their 70s, maybe they will be a little more open about sex and intimacy. Until then, however, there is not much one can do to bring conversations regarding sex among the elderly into the mainstream. Nor is it going to be considered appropriate to start discussing this openly with the elders at home. It would only make everyone uncomfortable.

However, if you have both of your parents living with you, what you can do is quietly and unobtrusively create a more conducive environment for them to find opportunities for intimacy. To begin with, you could ensure that they have a room to themselves so they have some privacy, and leave the rest up to them. You could subscribe to magazines that cater to the elder segment and hope that those magazines have articles covering various aspects of physical and emotional intimacy among senior citizens. You could also arrange for some holidays for just the two of them once in a while where they would be able to be together by themselves.

More importantly, you could try and not do some things. For example, in many families where there are multiple siblings ready to look after the parents, the siblings divvy up the parents' time, with one parent staying with one child for some time while the other parent goes and lives with another child. After a period, they are moved around so that eventually, over a year's time or so, all the children get to spend time with each of the parents. This is done with good intent but without taking into consideration how the parents might feel about being separated so callously.

If you have done this in your family, it may be time to reconsider your plans for your elders. See how you can ensure that both your parents are together when they move from one sibling to another. Better still, let them decide where they want to stay and when they would like to move elsewhere. And if they want to move into a retirement community, see if you can be supportive of that.

One other common practice in homes with elders is making the elders share the room with their grandchildren. If this is done because of space constraints, then everyone should take turns having the children share their room. The children could sleep in their parents' room on some days and in their grandparents' room on other days.

If this is done not because of space constraints but for other reasons, then this practice must be stopped completely. It is enough for the grandparents and the grandchildren to spend time and bond with each other during waking hours.

Help

If you come from a more progressive family, then do note that there are a few products in the market today that can make senior intimacy better. These include pills and gadgets that address issues relating to erectile dysfunction among men and lubricants to combat vaginal dryness common in postmenopausal women.

18

Dementia Care

Dementia is not the name for a single disease. It is an umbrella term for diseases and conditions in which there is a gradual but marked decline in cognitive capabilities, including memory. Alzheimer's is one common cause of dementia.

Memory loss is an early symptom. However, it must be remembered that some memory loss is normal as people age. Many elders worry unnecessarily because they misplace their glasses every now and then or sometimes forget why they entered a room. These incidents are not proof of the onset of dementia. We all forget things once in a while. However, if these incidents happen regularly or happen along with other symptoms, then it may be time to go and see a neurologist.

Dementia is progressive. However, it may be slowed down during the initial stages with medication and other non-medical interventions in some cases. In the long-term, unfortunately, there is no stopping or reversing it. It will gradually become worse and go through multiple stages before it can be finally termed 'full-blown', advanced, or end-stage when the elder will be unable to perform any activity properly.

As the brain is a complex machine, there is no way to predict exactly how the disease will progress, which faculties will get affected and in which order. Each case is likely to be unique, though there are definitely common traits.

For some, the deterioration may be slow while for others, the disease may progress rapidly. Memory loss is common, as is the inability to understand complex instructions. Some may display dramatic changes in behaviour and personality in complete contrast to their original selves. Some may become abusive and yet others may even become physically violent.

While dementia is a terminal illness, most people don't necessarily die of it. More often than not, other conditions and complications, undoubtedly exacerbated by dementia, are the cause of death.

What this means is that as a caregiver, you need to be prepared for a long road ahead and work consciously to make life easier for the person suffering from dementia and for yourself.

List of symptoms

Below are some of the common symptoms of dementia and suggestions on how you may be able to tackle them. These will undoubtedly test your patience, but if you remember the best in the person with dementia, you will be able to manage to maintain your composure and remain kind and caring throughout. Most people regret the harsh words they have spoken to their loved one during this period. So, watch what you say, for the loved one may not notice it, but your words will continue to ring in your own ears for a long, long time.

Memory loss

As mentioned earlier, one of the first signs of the onset of dementia is memory loss. During the initial stages, most often short-term memory gets affected while older memories may be retained. If an elder loved one complains about memory loss and is able to give examples of recent incidents, the chances are that they don't have dementia. Most dementia patients don't realize that they have actually forgotten something.

One common experience faced by many caregivers relates to the person with dementia forgetting instructions and then complaining about it. For example, you tell them that you are going to the neighbourhood pharmacy to get their medicines and that you should be back in ten minutes, and leave. Moments later, the elder calls a relative and complains that you are not there and they don't know anything about where you have gone and when you are likely to be back. In all probability, the relative then calls you in a panic and asks you why you have left the elder alone and gone gallivanting around town!

When such a thing happens, your immediate reaction might be to think that the elder one is creating trouble for you on purpose. However, the truth could very well be that the elder one completely forgot what you had said even before you were out of the door. That they selectively knew the most meddlesome relative to call and the correct phone number to dial can be all the more annoying, but that is also entirely consistent with dementia.

You could pre-empt this kind of situation in many ways. You could write a note and give it to the elder one or stick the note on the phone if you know they are going to make a beeline for it as soon as you are gone. You could also call the person they are most likely to call (if you know who that might be) and inform them about your going out and to keep the elder one occupied if they were to call. Basically, you need to figure out what is most likely to happen and take the necessary counter-measures. Experience, as always, is a great teacher.

Impaired judgement

Another common early symptom is loss of judgement. They might let strangers into the house or not let friends in because you have instructed them not to let anyone in. They might climb on to a chair or table to reach out for something kept in the loft, not realizing that they are no longer nimble enough to do that.

During the early days, before you have actually recognized or accepted that they have this condition, if they are mobile and going out on a regular basis, you may notice that they cross roads unsafely or drive rashly. Under such circumstances, it is best to gradually curtail their activities outside the house so that they are not a danger to themselves and to others.

This curtailing of freedom will not sit well with the elder and hence needs to be done kindly and gradually. If they want to go out, have someone accompany them. Hold their hand. If they object, tell them you are feeling a little dizzy instead of admonishing them. Get a driver or have someone else at home do the driving. Blame the increase in drunken drivers on the road if they ask why.

You know the person. You will figure out a way to get them to cooperate.

Difficulty in abstract thinking

You will notice that it gradually becomes more and more difficult for the elder loved one to follow long conversations and respond appropriately. They may also get angry and frustrated because they are unable to follow multiple instructions. Again, it is not that they are trying to be obtuse on purpose.

An easy way to avoid this is to give one instruction at a time. If you are taking them to a doctor, for example, you could first ask them to get dressed. Then you could ask them to wear their footwear. Once that is done, you could take them to the car and then ask them to get in. And so on. Once you do this a few times, it will become second nature to you. As their condition progresses, you may have to repeat the same instruction multiple times. But hopefully, by then you will be an expert at this, and having to parrot the same thing repeatedly will no longer cause your blood pressure to rise.

Faulty reasoning

Logical reasoning also gets impaired. They may argue about even the simplest things or they may act illogically. For example, they may wear their shoes first and then try to put on their socks. Pointing it out may make them argumentative. Arguing with them or trying to convince them that they are wrong will usually not work. Somewhere at the back of their mind, they may also know that they are wrong and so, arguing with them might only add to their frustration.

During these times, you should just hold your peace for a while. They usually forget the reason for the argument soon afterwards. Once they have quietened down, you can give them simple instructions and move them along.

Inappropriate behaviour

As the condition progresses, it is possible that they display inappropriate behaviour. It is important to remember that they are not in their senses and are not in control of their actions. It is also equally important to keep in mind that these are not to be construed as repressed thoughts being acted out. What they do may be no reflection of who they were or what their attitudes used to be when they were healthy and well.

If some of this inappropriate behaviour is directed at the hired help or visitors, it may be misconstrued and can lead to unnecessary complications and friction. It is important to sensitize outsiders about what to expect and how to react if they were to face such behaviour. Especially in the case of a male patient and female hired help, abuse or sexually explicit gestures can have serious repercussions, as one can imagine.

It is not unheard of to find the hired help retaliating by physically abusing the patient when no one else is around. This happens usually when family members leave the hired help to fend for themselves. However, if family members intervene on behalf of the hired help and bear the brunt of most of the abuse and take the side of the hired help (unobtrusively, if necessary) whenever possible, then maybe the hired help would not get too frustrated or plan retaliation.

Anyway, as a policy, it is important that you are unfailingly courteous and kind to the hired help so that they remain happy and, in turn, are caring towards your loved one even when you are not around. Also, it helps to have a CCTV camera installed.

Loss of communication skills

Even in the initial stages, you will find that there are long pauses when they are obviously searching for words to express their thoughts. This can worsen as days go by and as the illness progresses. At some stage, they may not be able to even complete their sentences properly. Be patient and wait it out. If it is important, you can try to bring up the topic again after some time. If it is not important, just let it be.

Disorientation with respect to time and place

Another noticeable symptom is that the person suffering from dementia often forgets where they are. They may also lose track of time to the extent that they may not even know which year it is! One of the common requests you will get from them is to be taken home even though they are already at home. This could be because they remember their childhood home better than their current one. It is mostly no use telling them that they are already home. It is easier on everyone if you just tell them that you will take them home as soon as you are done with your work. That can usually calm them down.

Due to the disorientation, persons with dementia tend to wander off and get lost. It is important to ensure that they are always accompanied. There are also a lot of wearable gadgets available in the market that use GPS to help you keep track of your elders.

Additionally, remember that dementia is nothing to be ashamed of. Keep your neighbours in the loop so they are also on the lookout. If by chance the care recipient gives you the slip, a neighbour or friend will be there to stop them from going too far away.

Gait, motor and balance problems

Some of the biggest complications resulting from dementia are the falls, bruises and broken bones that result from the loss of balance that some of the patients suffer. For many people, loss of balance is also one of the early signs. So, if you notice memory lapses along with loss of balance, change in gait and/or inability to hold a pen, doorknobs and railings, you should immediately get them evaluated. As the disease progresses, these become more pronounced. Towards the end, many persons with dementia find it difficult even to get up and stand unaided.

You can refer to Chapter 14 titled 'A Safe and Secure Environment for Elders' to get tips on how you can reduce the chances of falls. If falls and broken bones are prevented, the person can remain active for a long time, making life easier for everyone. If, on the other hand, a fall results in a pelvic fracture, for example, this will entail hospitalization, which can lead to further difficulties and, eventually, instead of a mobile care recipient, you might end up with one who is bedridden.

Neglect of personal care and safety

As the dementia sufferer withdraws from the world, they tend to lose self-awareness as well. Consequently, they start to neglect how they look, forget to brush their teeth, wash hands and wash themselves. Hygiene takes a big hit. Again, the complications resulting from the neglect of personal care can be severe. Injuries, infection, food poisoning, urinary tract infections and several other issues can crop up as a result.

Thankfully, as they are with their family, proper care and a good hygiene routine can keep such problems at bay. Think of them as children. That way, it will become a habit for you to check if they are following all the important hygiene practices, from brushing their teeth to washing hands properly with soap. If they allow, have a same-sex member of the family or hired help to supervise and assist them in their daily hygiene activities.

Hallucinations, paranoia, agitation

At advanced stages of the disease, hallucinations, paranoia and agitation are common. Some might talk continuously while others may address people who are not even there. Some can also become highly suspicious. Though this can be quite disturbing for family members, it is important that they don't take it personally. It is the disease that is making them behave in such a way.

One elderly gentleman suffering from dementia insisted on checking all his bank passbooks every day. He was convinced that his only son, who was the primary caregiver (and sole inheritor), was out to swindle him of all his money and property. Another lady complained to every visitor that her daughter-in-law was poisoning her and stealing all her diamond jewellery.

The best way to handle such situations is either to accede to their demand, as was done in the former case (the elder gentleman became peaceful for the rest of the day, once he had reviewed his passbooks), or to ignore them, as would be ideal in the latter example, and move on. Arguments and fights can only make things worse.

Incontinence management

You may have already read Chapter 13 titled 'Incontinence Management'. This note is about something specific to persons with dementia. Some of them have very fidgety hands. So, routinely during the course of the night, they end up pulling the tabs off the nappy-type diapers that are recommended for people with heavy incontinence. This can result in the diaper falling off and urine spilling all over their clothes and bed.

To save you a lot of cleaning work, if your loved one has the habit of pulling off their diaper, switch to pull-on diapers. These are more difficult to remove, though they may be less absorbent. Alternatively, you could get them to wear the thin, disposable mesh panties that are available in the market, over the diaper. These will hold the diaper in place and prevent the person with dementia from removing their diaper.

Activities for delaying progression

A lot of activities can slow down the progression of the disease. Social interaction, games based on words and numbers, card games and strategy games—all provide different brain exercises that are proven to be effective.

In addition, using one's non-dominant hand for routine tasks, learning a new language, learning to play a musical instrument, or even listening to music can lead to better cognition and memory retention.

19

Activities for Seniors

As a family caregiver, you need to ensure that the elders at home are occupied and active. Doing so will ensure that they are healthy, happy and active for a long time.

As people age, many of their favourite activities become progressively more difficult to do. That game of badminton, those long treks, the overseas trips to be with their grandchildren—all gradually become too taxing for their body, no matter what their spirit may want.

However, these activities cannot all be given up totally as the benefits of these physical and social activities are undeniable, both in terms of physical well-being as well as mental health. As many studies have shown, exercise and social interactions can:

- Extend the period of active life.
- Improve physical health, maintain balance, slow down muscle degeneration, and retain strength and stamina.
- Boost the immune system.
- Help improve or retain good brain function.
- Maintain emotional health.
- Provide better sleep.

In order to take advantage of these benefits, it is necessary to find suitable activities, both physical and mental, to replace those that are no longer possible.

This chapter aims to list out a few possible activities for people in various conditions.

Activities for the fit

Elders who are still agile and fit can continue to do many of their favourite activities, though they may have to reduce the frequency and the intensity of the activity. They can also plan carefully to ensure that they do not overstrain or injure themselves, as recovery can be slow and painful.

Travel

While travelling, a few simple checks, requests and changes in schedule can go a long way in making travel comfortable and enjoyable. Look for comfortable travel times, and book trains and planes that depart and arrive at decent hours. If there is bus travel involved, especially in India, ensure that they are short enough to not require bathroom breaks. Overnight bus journeys can be hard on the bladder. Alternatively, get them to practice using a diaper in the sanctuary of their homes so that they are ready in an emergency. If long flights are involved, ensure that they use compression stockings during the journey. These are graduated stockings that prevent Deep Vein Thrombosis, a very painful condition that can cause serious complications.

While booking hotel and resort rooms, it is good to request for ground-floor rooms. Additionally, check if all areas of the hotel/resort, including the restaurant and recreational areas, are accessible without necessitating the use of the stairs.

If the travellers have dietary restrictions, then check if the restaurant is capable of meeting their dietary needs. Are there sugar-free desserts? Low-salt meals? Vegan substitutes?

Physical sports and exercise

Contact sports and those that are high-impact will gradually have to be given up. Sports like badminton and tennis can put a lot of strain, especially on the knees.

These activities may be replaced with lower impact ones such as walking, golf, swimming, cycling, yoga and even dancing. Aerobics, cardio and resistance training exercises can also be included in the regimen, preferably under the guidance of a qualified instructor who knows what they are doing.

Activities for the mobility-challenged

Even for those elders who need the support of mobility aids—whether walking sticks or wheelchairs—there are activities that can be safely practiced.

Hydrotherapy

Also called hydropathy, this is the practice of doing exercises in a swimming pool. A typical pool meant for hydrotherapy will be about three to four feet deep uniformly with conveniently placed railings. Elders can hold the railings and walk or run or do other simple exercises. The water in the pool provides more resistance than the air, thereby making the muscles work harder while simultaneously cushioning all the impact. The buoyancy also lets weak legs bear the bodyweight better.

Hydrotherapy is especially good for people with arthritis.

Chair yoga

There are a lot of classes which teach specific yogasanas that have been modified to enable one to do yoga while seated. The Internet is full of videos made specifically with elders in mind. Thanks to yoga's recent re-emergence and popularity, you may also find a yoga teacher in your locality.

Activities to keep your brain ticking

Just as the body requires exercises to keep fit, so does the brain. There are a lot of activities that can keep the brain active and help elders defer or slow down mental illnesses such as Parkinson's, Alzheimer's and other forms of dementia.

Reading and socializing are two of the best ways to keep the brain happy and active. In addition, many board games are available which provide challenges at various degrees of difficulty. Crossword puzzles, Sudoku and numerous other games and brain teasers are available as apps on phones and similar gadgets.

Just like the different muscles in our body, the brain also has different areas for different kinds of processing. So, the more diverse our range of mental activities, the better the chances of keeping mental illnesses at bay.

Some activities such as learning a new language, using the non-dominant hand to perform routine tasks and learning to play a new instrument are also brain exercises with proven benefits.

Conclusion

As already noted elsewhere in the book, family caregivers are among the most unappreciated of people. It is not intentional on the part of the others, as you probably realize, but nevertheless quite true. So, it would be thoughtless if even a book on family caregiving such as this one had only one chapter devoted to the well-being of the caregiver. So, here is one more chapter—this time dedicated to the future well-being of you, dear, kind-hearted caregiver.

Let us begin with a sobering thought—much as we may not want to think about it, in a decade or three, some of us caregivers may very well be care recipients ourselves. Not all of us, of course. In fact, most of us will probably live to a ripe old age and die peacefully in our sleep or after a very brief period of illness. However, going by past records, for about

10 per cent of us, the path to our end may not be as simple or trouble-free.

Most people don't properly plan for their later years, except perhaps financially. But as people who have had a close look at the ravages wrought by old age, it would be unconscionable if we don't use our hard-earned experience to analyze and take necessary action to mitigate at least some of the problems senior citizens are likely to face in the near future.

So, in this concluding chapter, let us look ahead and see how we can make use of the next few decades to shape our future world into a much better place for ourselves and other elders.

The future is definitely going to be different. Some longevity scientists even go so far as to say that the first person to live to be 150 years old has already been born. If that is true, many of us are going to live much longer than our parents and grandparents. What is not clear, however, is how healthy we will be during that extended period. Much as we would like to believe in science following science fiction, it is unlikely that we would have conquered death and disease completely by then.

Thus, unless medical science defies all expectations and advances even faster than it is doing now, we will all have to confront at least some of the issues associated with ageing faced by our care recipients today. Our faculties will grow weaker, our bodies will suffer from wear and tear and our minds may not remain as sharp as they were in our younger days. Most of us, at some point in time, will need some amount of support to carry out the activities of daily living, even if it just means somebody will have to cook and clean for us.

On the positive side, if we continue along the current trajectory, some improvements are bound to accrue, making life better for us in our old age. For example, there will definitely be more retirement communities and palliative care institutions around with more experience to help us. Undoubtedly, self-diagnostic tools would have improved significantly, making monitoring one's vitals as easy as using the mobile phone today. In conjunction with telemedicine and video conferencing (which are already seeing an explosion, thanks primarily to the Covid-19 pandemic), this would make consulting a doctor from the comfort of our homes, a safe and painless process.

Of course, not everything would have changed for the better. One area where we may be worse off is in the area of family caregiving. Large families with four, five or more children are a thing of the past and, in all probability, we each have only one or, at most, two children of our own. If we are lucky, they may be living close to us, but in all likelihood, their career would have taken them far away from us, which will mean that we are likely to be on our own in our later years.

This is where our experience in caregiving should be able to help us. If we all put our minds to it, maybe we can make changes, both at a personal level and on a larger scale, to shape for ourselves a better future. Who knows—maybe if we can all work together, we may even be able to lobby, coax and cajole the powers-that-be into making this country of ours more senior-friendly in the future.

Given below are some of the activities you can put into action. This is by no means an exhaustive list as we all know that there are more things we can do to improve life in India than we can shake a stick at.

Personal changes

There are many aspects of our physical and mental health that we cannot control. A stroke, for example, that can leave one incapacitated cannot always be predicted or averted. Similarly, we still don't know what causes dementia and who is likely to be affected.

However, there are many other aspects of health that are largely under our control. According to doctors, with discipline, a proper diet and regular exercise, we can all hope to stave off lifestyle diseases such as Type-II diabetes, some forms of hypertension and heart diseases, as well as diseases associated with excessive smoking and drinking.

Another aspect that is likely—though not always—to be under our control is our weight. Many of us have personal experience in this area and know first-hand how even regular tasks such as changing diapers become significantly more difficult when the care recipient is bulky.

Similarly, we know from collective experience that bedridden people who accept their situation and remain cheerful are easier to look after than those who are bitter and complain about their undeniably unfair fate.

Taking all our learnings into consideration, it may be a good idea to make a few lifestyle changes starting now in order to improve our chances for a better and healthier future. Here's a list to begin with:

- Meet a professional dietician and chalk out a good diet for ourselves. Depending on our preferences, constraints and dietary habits, the dietician will be able to outline the kind of foods and their proportions we should include in our diet.
- Get the help of a professional trainer or a yoga teacher, join a gym or plan our own exercise regimen. Depending on our age and current health conditions, our exercise regimen should include a judicious mix of cardiovascular exercises, strength-building workouts as well as routines to improve our flexibility and balance. If we are overweight, we should ensure that our exercise

regimen is tailored to help us reach the right weight for our height and age.

- Include meditation and breathing exercises into our day-to-day activities.
- Those of us who are smokers should try giving up on it entirely as more and more studies are showing that there is no safe level of smoking. Those of us who drink regularly should try and gradually cut down on our intake.
- As a caregiver, we have learnt to accept the mortality of our loved ones. It is time for us to reconcile with our own mortality as well. This will hold us in good stead whether we find ourselves in the unfortunate situation of being dependent on someone else or not. After all, death is inevitable and we will all face it one day or the other.

Be a changemaker in your community

We may not realize this now, but the experience we have gained as caregivers is extremely valuable and quite hard to come by. No school or institute teaches a course on family caregiving, nor would a theoretical course come anywhere near teaching us what we have learnt in real life while on the job.

So, while we may all want to get back to our lives once our stint as a family caregiver ends, it may be a good idea to use our experience for the benefit of others and possibly our own future selves. We could:

- *Start a self-help group:* After all, no one understands a caregiver better than another caregiver. It could be a group that meets in person or online on a regular basis, or it could be a website or podcast that helps caregivers connect, share their experiences, or even vent in a safe environment where they will not be misunderstood or judged. Such self-help groups go a long way in staving off depression and the feeling that life is just passing us by.

- *Start a companionship group:* Many elders living by themselves suffer from depression brought on by a lack of social interaction. Those of us who are physically active, no matter what age, can make some time to provide companionship to elders while simultaneously enabling their caregivers to have some 'me' time.

- *Collate relevant information:* We know the kind of emergency and non-emergency information and services that are required for a household with senior citizens. We could take one area, maybe where we currently live, for example, and collate all such pieces of information and disseminate that through a website, WhatsApp group or even the local newspaper. Some of the data could include contact details of pharmacies, hospitals, doctors that do home visits, nursing services, other home healthcare services, ambulance services, oxygen providers as well as barbers that do house calls, companies that deliver vegetables, people who provide home-cooked meals and so on.

- *Teach elders new skills:* Many elders continue to struggle to use their computers. Those of us who are conversant with using computers could help elders to learn how to use net banking services safely to pay their bills online, use the various social networking sites, as well as use tools like Skype, WhatsApp and Zoom, to name a few, to connect with family and friends on a regular basis.

Work on a larger scale

India as a country is unfortunately not very senior-friendly. If one were to search online for 'safest country for elders', one would find reports from hundreds of independent studies conducted by NGOs and magazines, and invariably, in each of these reports, India is ranked somewhere in the middle. This is quite sad, given how much as a culture we revere the elderly in our country.

This is an area in which we can make a huge impact. Many of us caregivers are also professionals. Among us are lawyers, judges, doctors, architects, engineers,

IAS officers, filmmakers, writers, journalists, politicians and people from every other walk of life. We could all use our individual skills and knowledge to effect dramatic changes to how India takes care of its elders. Here are some ideas:

- *Accessibility*: Public areas in India are uniformly senior-unfriendly. Whether it is the local bank or post office, or parks, malls or theatres, they are usually very difficult to navigate for an elderly person. We could lobby our local bodies to build ramps, provide preferential parking spaces and other special facilities that can make life easier for elders. One ramp at a time, we can change the country for the elders today and for ourselves in the future.

- *Concessions for elders*: Discounts for train and air travel, a small increase in interest rates on fixed deposits and rebate on income tax are some of the few special concessions that senior citizens benefit from in India. There is a lot more that can be done in this area. For example, the lobbying organization AARP in the US is constantly working closely with many private organizations, from restaurants to theatres to malls, to provide special, subsidized rates to senior citizens. In many countries, entry tickets at zoos, museums and other places of entertainment are subsidized for senior citizens. It is time that Indian senior citizens form a powerful lobbying organization of their own that aims to make the lives of elders safer, more secure and comfortable.

- *Start a business*: Of course, not everything needs to be in the form of free service. For those with a business mindset, any establishment that can provide a valuable service and make life easier for elders would also be a great idea. There are not that many such businesses in India and as a greenfield investment, and with such a large target segment, chances of succeeding are quite high.

As seasoned caregivers, we are in the best position to envisage a future India that is more friendly towards senior citizens.

Come, let us join hands and make the vision of a more senior-friendly India a reality.